MEN'S HAIR

MEN'S HAIR

by George Roberson

with Leonard McGill and Carol Tonsing

Designed by Jay Purvis

Rawson Associates : New York

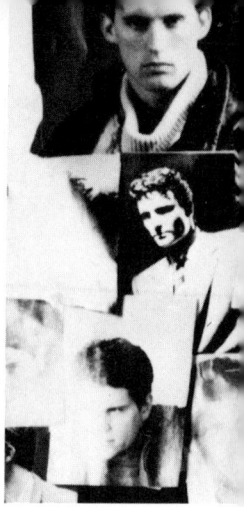

Library of Congress Cataloging in Publication Data

Roberson, George.
  Men's hair.

  Includes index.
  1. Hair—Care and hygiene. 2. Grooming for men.
I. McGill, Leonard, 1956–   . II. Tonsing, Carol, 1941–. III. Title.
IV. Title:
Men's hair.
RL91.R63   1985   646.7′24′088041   84-42541
ISBN 0-89256-275-7

Published simultaneously in Canada by McClelland and Stewart Ltd.
Packaged by Rapid Transcript
Composition by Folio Graphics Co., Inc.

Designed by Jay Purvis and Randy Dunbar
Printed and bound by Fairfield Graphics, Fairfield, Pennsylvania
First Edition

All photographs, with the exception of those indicated, were taken by
Gregory Cannon, copyright © 1984 by Cannon Studios, Inc.

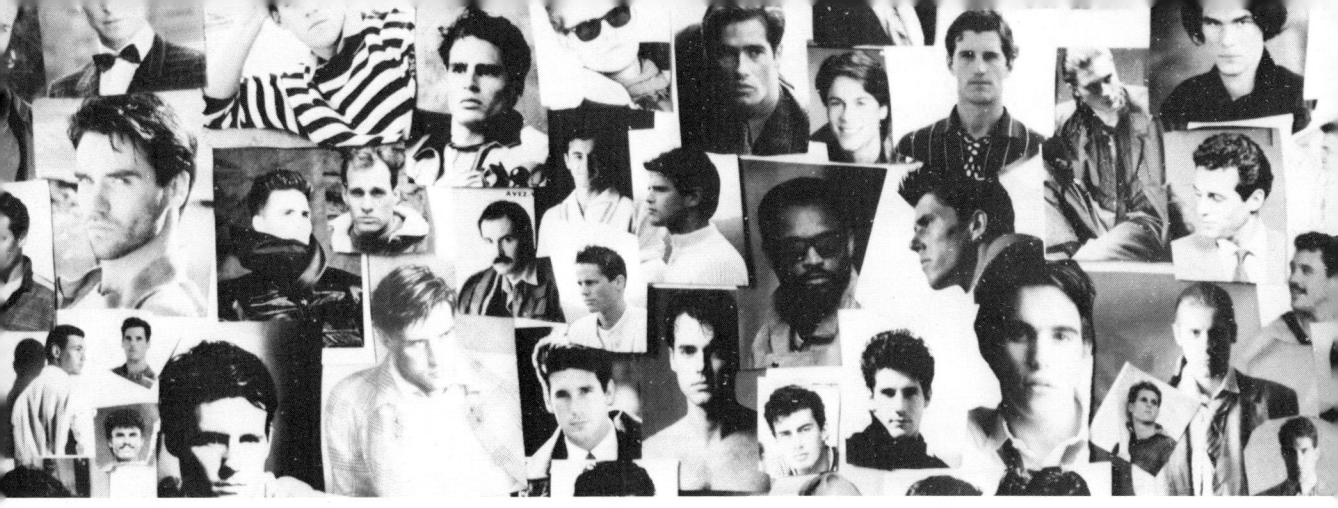

I would like to thank

Gregory Cannon for his beautiful photographs;
My literary agents, Connie Clausen and Guy Kettelhack;
Adele Scheele, who first encouraged me to write this book;
My dear friend Charlie Springman, who is a constant source of inspiration and support;
Kris Evans for her love and encouragement;
Tracy Thompson, who makes me laugh even at the most grueling moments;
Susanna Weiss, my exercise coach, for helping me regroup my body and soul;
Mark Garbin for his computer wizardry;
Jon and Jude Kane for beautiful illustrations;
Randy Dunbar for dedicated design work;
My family for their love.

Special thanks to Jay Purvis, an inspiring friend and talented visual designer, who has worked with me on *Men's Hair* from the very beginning. His book design is vital in conveying the message and instruction of *Men's Hair.*

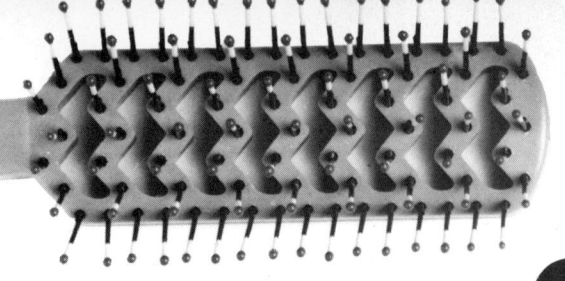

Contents

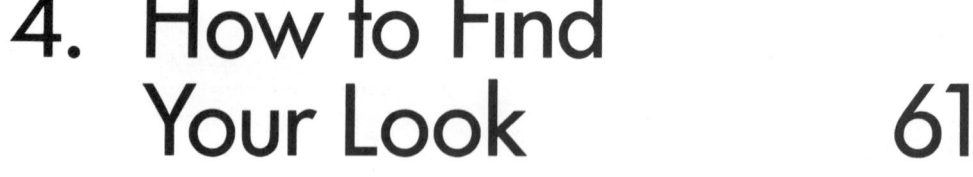

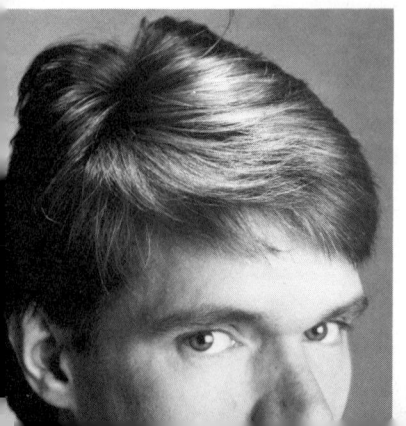

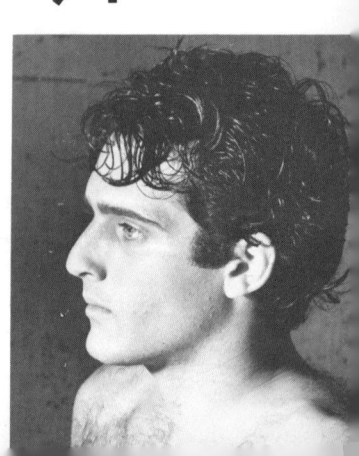

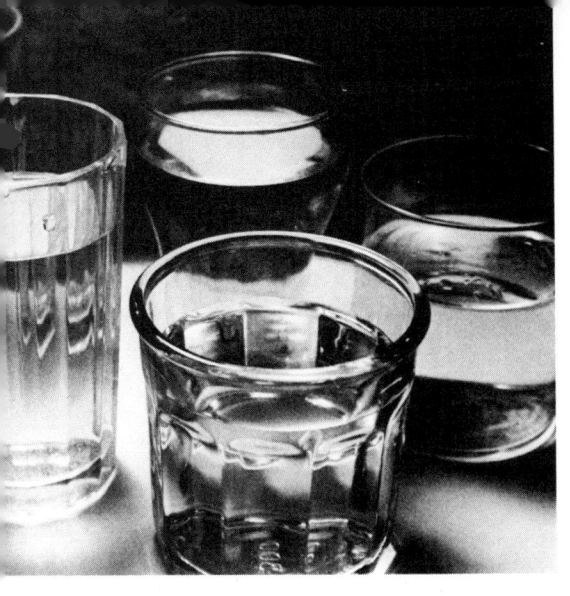
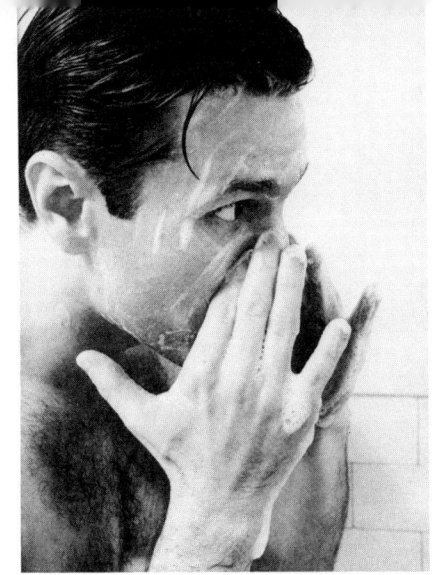

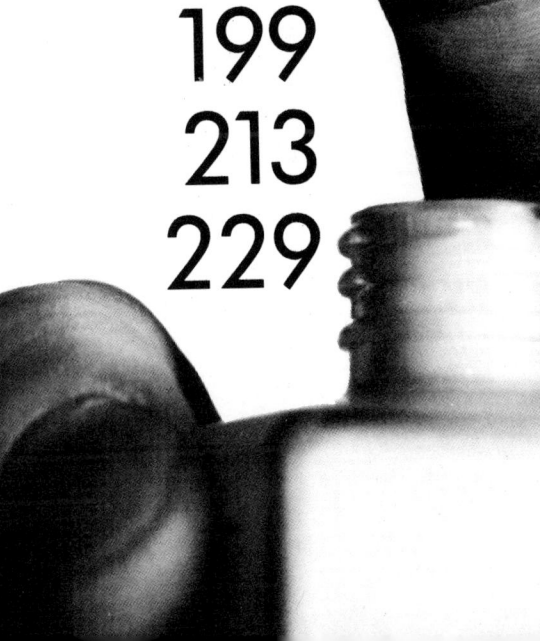

I am a hair stylist and I love my work. I feel a sense of power when I transform a man who thought of himself as a loser in the looks department into a winner. Many men are unaware of the impact the right hair can give them and have exempted themselves from what they see as an unmanly preoccupation with their looks. I hope to change this with *Men's Hair*. Taking care of yourself and looking your best is for all people, not for any particular gender. Why not be open to new ideas? Help yourself to look your best and get a boost in all areas of your life.

1.

HAIR POWER

Good-Looking Hair Can Give You the Look of Success

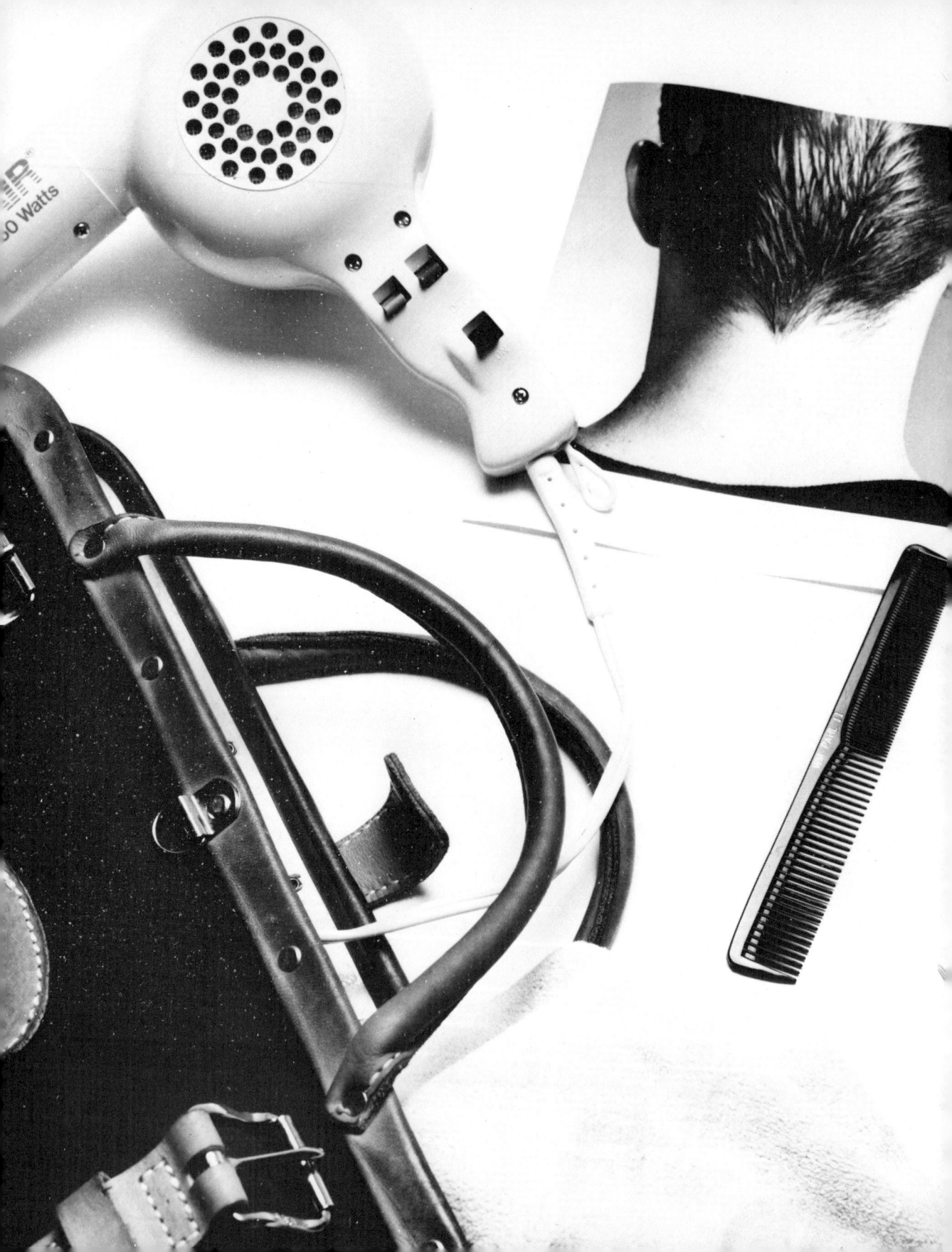

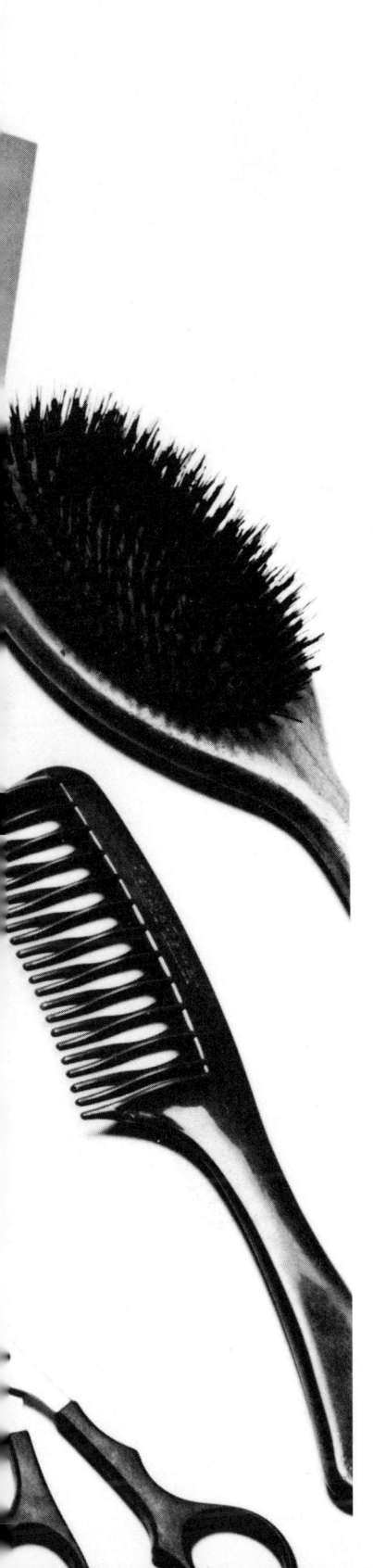

The Key to the Look of Success

Your hair is the most important aspect of your good looks. It immediately influences how you appear to others. Your hair is so powerful it can make or break that crucial good first impression.

What do you think of first when you conjure up the appearance of President Ronald Reagan, Walter Mondale, Jesse Jackson, Tom Selleck, Pernell Roberts of "Trapper John," Fidel Castro, Albert Einstein, Robert Redford? For better or for worse, it's their hair. Would many people recognize Castro without a beard, Selleck without a moustache? Can you imagine a dark-haired Redford, a balding Reagan?

The right haircut makes an instant impact, even though it might not—and in most cases should not—call attention to itself. (Actors always use their hairstyle to help create an image or portray a character.) What's important is that good-looking hair can give you the boost of confidence, the look of success that can help you in business; it can give you a smooth, elegant, self-assured appearance that will open doors for you socially; it can give you a virile, sexy, romantic dash that spices up your love life. You can use your hair to play up your physical assets, play down your flaws, reinforce the mood you want to project.

The best news is that everyone can have great-looking hair. This is true even if a man's hair is thinning. So why have men been giving this vital part of their looks short shrift for so long?

They've been leaving it in the hands of others, taking it for granted (until it starts falling out). They follow styles in hair willy-nilly, with little regard to how they relate to their facial features or their lifestyle. They're unaware of the many options available to help their hair reach its maximum potential.

These days we've been paying new attention to the rest of our bodies. We're dressing for success, to be more competitive in the business world. We're working out to get the bodies we want. But most of us are still not using the one feature that can make our most dramatic statement and over which we have the most control: our hair.

People notice your hair before they notice your beautifully fitted suit or impressive physique. And if your hairstyle is *wrong*, no tailor or gym coach can remedy the situation. Give it the importance it deserves!

Women have always known the power of beautiful hair. They get curlers when they're five years old. We get baseball caps. They get admired for long golden curls or neat pigtails. We get dragged to the barbershop to have our curls lopped off.

I've worked with hundreds of men: television personalities on ABC's "Good Morning America," top fashion models in national ad campaigns, and average men like those you'll see in this book. One thing has been clear: Give a man a great look with the right haircut, beard, moustache, and skin care (whichever he needs) and he'll finally relax and feel good about himself.

Give yourself that and *you* will, too!

Bringing Out Your Strong Points—
Joe from Atlanta

Joe from Atlanta grew his hair long in his teens as an act of rebellion. As he grew older, he refused to cut it—it was too much a part of who he was, said Joe.

Joe had a great body and a strong jaw, but who noticed them under all that hair? When he moved to New York, I convinced him it was time to let his natural assets come out from under.

●**As a general rule:** Short hair will show off a good physique. That's the reason those oiled men who glisten on the cover of bodybuilding magazines always forsake the Samson look for a shorter cut that will show off the face, neck, shoulders, and entire upper body.

It took some coaxing, but I finally cut Joe's brown, coarse hair short on the sides and back, leaving a bit of tousled length on top for interest and to elongate his wide face.

The result: Joe said he felt differently about himself—more assertive, proud of his strong bone structure, and delighted to show off those hours of work in the gym. (Of course, a different haircut can make any man feel different. But the *right* haircut will add muscle to his image!) What's more, his hair now suits his new, confident lifestyle.

Harmonizing Hair and Body—
Allen the Singer

Allen, an aspiring singer/dancer, feels he could fill Radio City Music Hall with his voice. He was far less sure of his appearance. Before he came to

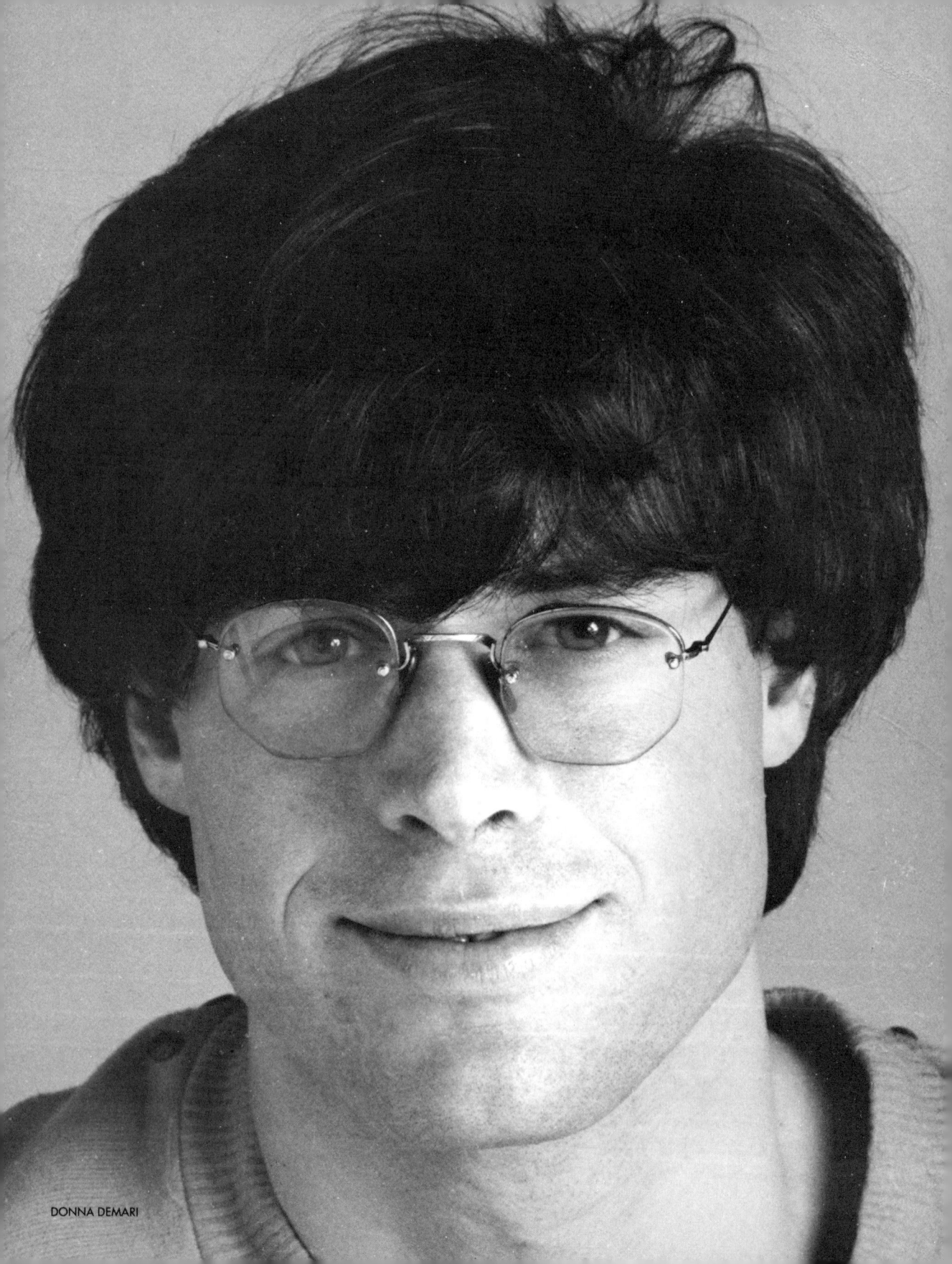

DONNA DEMARI

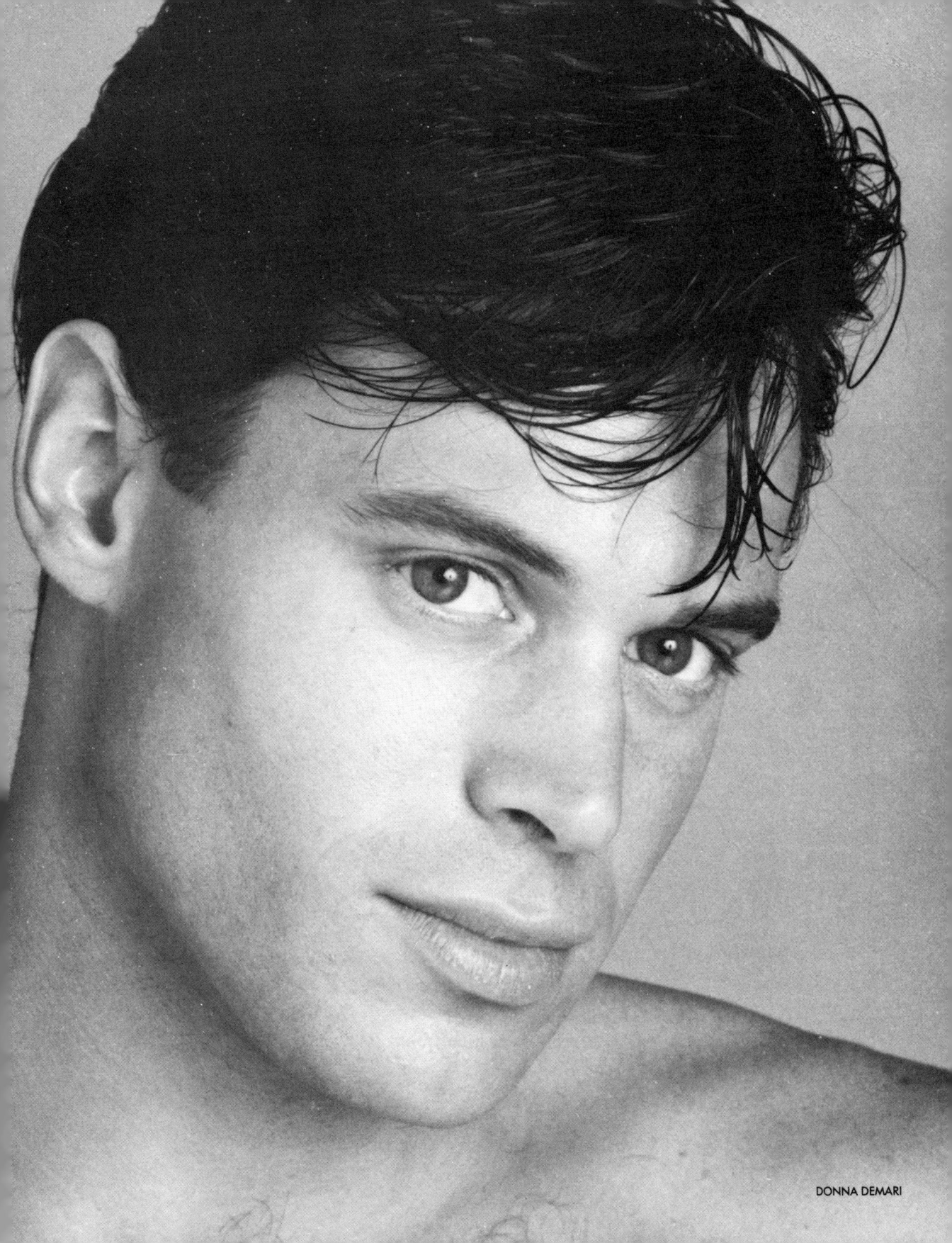

DONNA DEMARI

me, he had gone through life thinking his head looked too big, worried about the effect of his appearance on his career.

I saw immediately that his head size was *not* the problem. His features were large and very strong. With his very short hairstyle, they virtually leaped off his face.

● **As a general rule:** A short haircut makes the facial features jump out, become very pronounced. This is good for a rather undistinguished, undefined face that needs projection. But it's overpowering for someone with dramatic, large features (unless you deliberately want to play them up).

I encouraged Allen to let his hair grow and to stop blow-drying it. As his hair reached medium length, a natural wave appeared. The wave and the new length softened his features and made his head seem softer and more in proportion to his body.

The result: For the first time in his life, Allen felt really good about his appearance. He learned that his large features could be sized down by the right haircut and brought into a harmonious new proportion integrating his head with the rest of his body.

I believe the right hairstyle literally can change your life for the better. Men who were uneasy and frustrated about their self-image become positive and more assertive when they get a new, better look. And regardless of how much hair you have or what condition or style it is in now, you can use it to give you a powerful, sexier, more flattering look.

The point: If you look your best, you will feel more confident in every other aspect of your life. You can then relax, enjoy yourself, and take care of

John's Saturday Night Fever look is now dated. The stiff, too-perfect blow-dry style smacks of the '70s. Today's styles need more movement and freedom.

John's Urban Cowboy beard gives him outdoor appeal and brings out a new rugged dimension to his personality.

In Staying Alive, his hairstyle has short sides, a longer top. It's a current look.

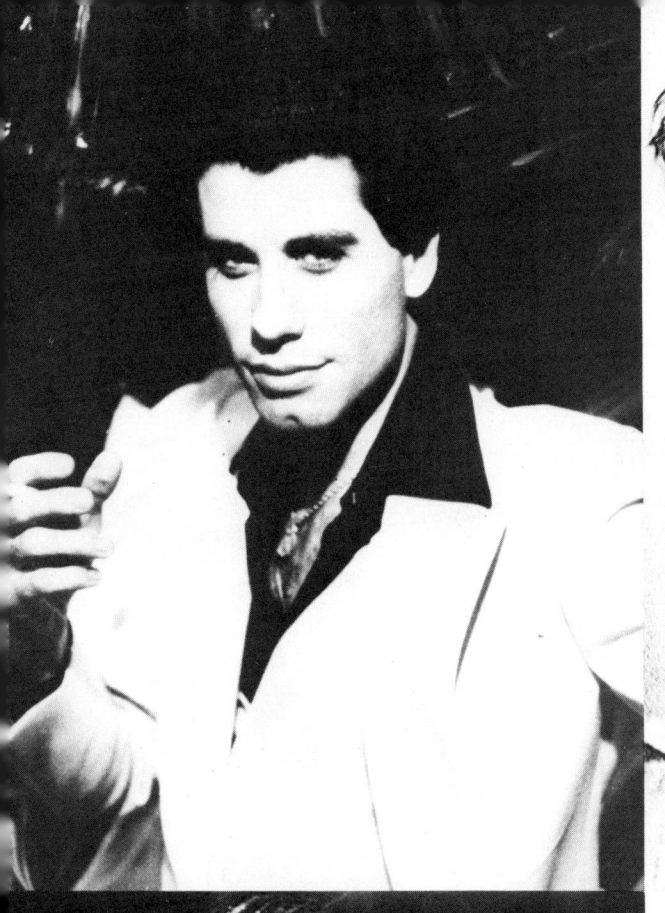

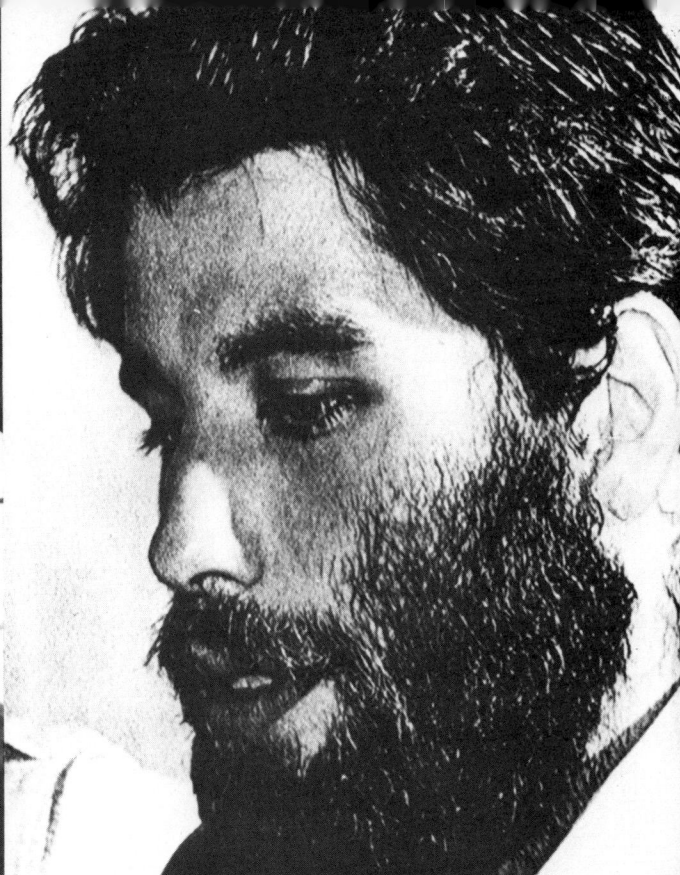

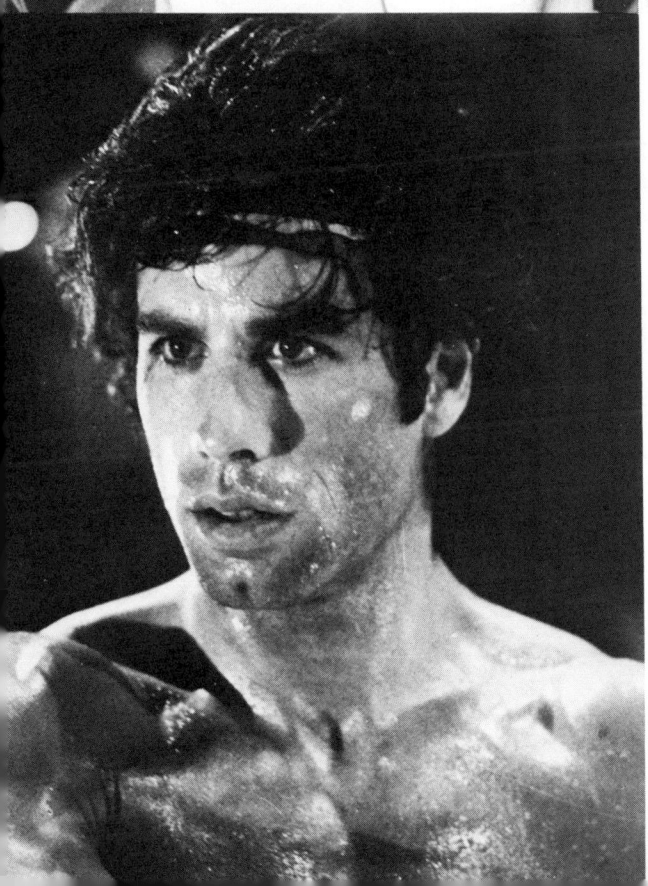

Different and distinct hairstyles give John Travolta a chameleon quality. Remember Vinnie Barbarino?

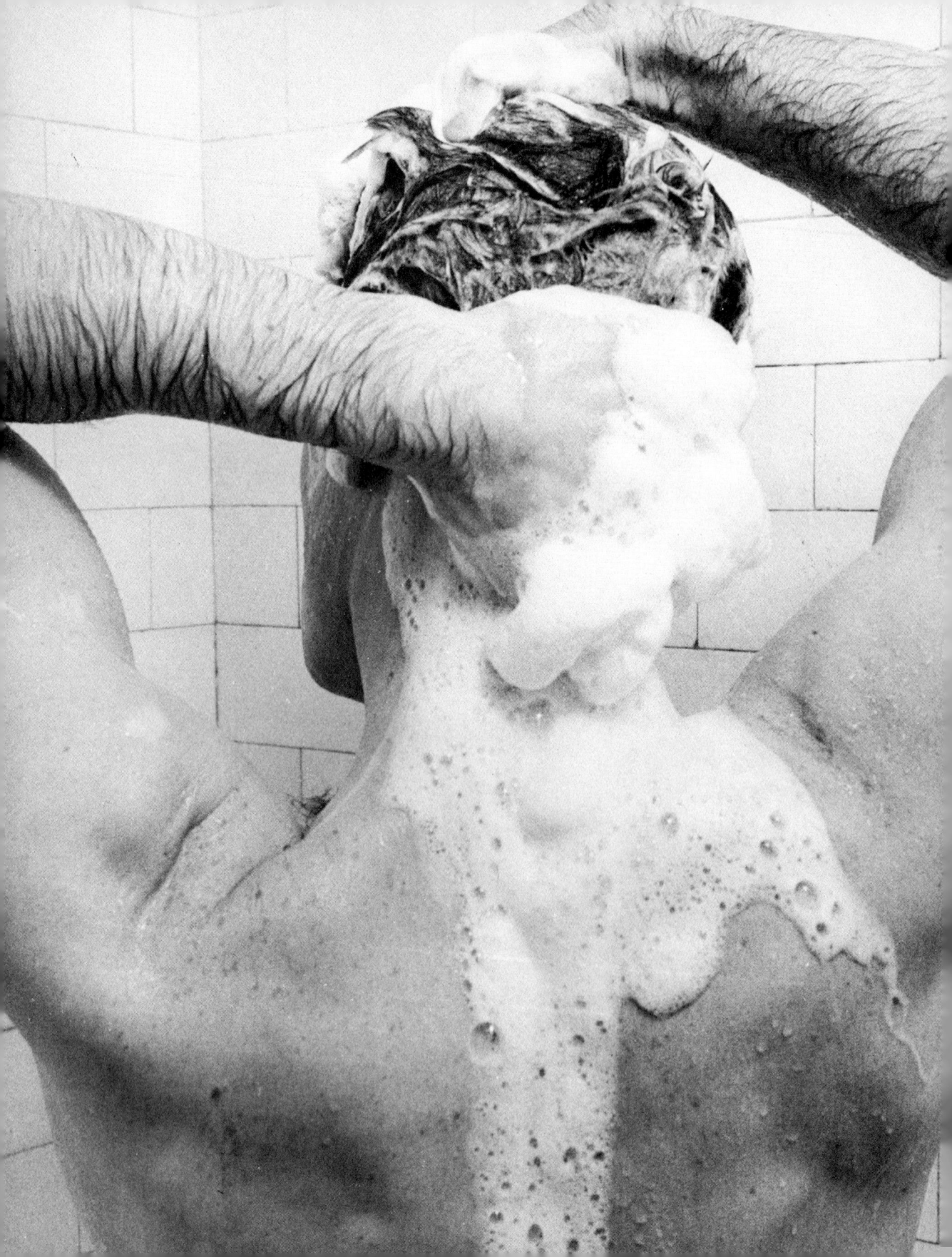

the other business at hand, sure that your looks are doing their very best work for you.

Versatile Hair—Switch, Don't Settle

Once you get the right cut, you don't have to settle for just one look. Hair is versatile. You don't dress the same for a country weekend as you do for a corporate meeting. You don't have to wear office hair every waking moment, either. One hairstyle can fit *all* the roles you have to play.

Let's say you wear a standard businessman's haircut—something like that of Lee Iacocca, chairman of Chrysler. Not too long. Not too short. Neat, side-parted, with a dab of holding cream (such as Brylcreem) rubbed in. When the weekend rolls around, here's how to have a more relaxed outdoors look.

Take a shower, shampooing out the Brylcreem. Use only a drop of creme rinse, just enough to give your hair shine and manageability. Then just towel your head and shake it. With your fingers only, *push* your hair into shape and let it dry naturally. Easy? You bet!

The point: Every man's hair can have at least two different moods.

One of the wonders of men's hair is that, chameleonlike, it can change dramatically to fit your activities, your moods, even the seasons. Sometimes it feels great to skip the morning shave and hair brushing and greet the sun with your hair looking as comfortably disheveled as a pair of flannel pajamas. Then again, if you'll be dining at a restaurant requiring you to wear a jacket and tie, you'll want to use a blow dryer or hair groomer to put and keep your hair in its proper place.

Give yourself the feeling of a wake-up shower and shampoo to begin your day fresh.

21

We dress differently in winter than we do in summer. And, as with a wool coat or cotton pants, our hair can change with the temperature, too. I like longer hair in winter, with maybe a short beard and moustache. When warmer weather comes, show off your athletic body with a cool, short cut that's virtually maintenance free.

Working with Your Hair

Everyone has a look that works for him, makes him feel confident and terrific. The trick is to find it. Once you do, there is no stopping you from fully realizing your hair's potential.

Say you have thick, bushy hair that you try to calm down every day. After your shower, you style it with a brush and hair spray. That's not *really* using your hair's potential. Try working *with* it instead. Have your stylist give you a soft haircut (like Joe from Atlanta) that's short on the sides and in back, so it will stay in place naturally. Now, instead of a brush and hair spray, you can shape your hair by running your fingers through it. It should just fall into the proportions you and your stylist have agreed upon.

The point: Get to know your hair, and don't underestimate its potential.

You're in Control

So much of how your hair looks depends on how much you know about it. Once you know your hair, you control it. It is simply a matter of learning. You already know much more than you realize.

As you read this guide—the culmination of hundreds of hours of my work on hundreds of

Graphs like the one below represent responses to my questionnaire. You'll find them all through the book.

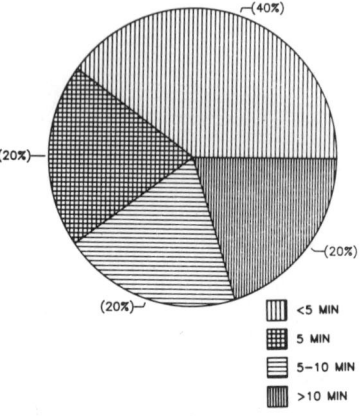

(40%)

(20%)

(20%)

(20%)

(20%)

▨ <5 MIN
▥ 5 MIN
▤ 5–10 MIN
▦ >10 MIN

Men's Hair questionnaires were sent to men throughout the country. I asked men about all aspects of their hair: care, daily maintenance, products used, how long between haircuts, etc. I also asked them about their favorite and least favorite facial and body features, their shaving routines, and if they were satisfied with their shave.

Among the other questions asked were for men's opinions favoring and against such controversial subjects as hair replacement, permanent waving, hair coloring, and makeup for men.

MEN'S HAIR

1. How often do you have your hair cut?

   About every two months

2. How often do you shampoo?

   Every day

3. Do you have a regular barber or stylist?

   No

4. Do you get compliments on your hair?

5. Do you know the difference between a finishing rinse and a conditioner? If yes, explain...

6. What features of your face do you like the most? Dislike?

7. Describe the texture, color and amount of your hair....

8. Do you use a grooming product on your hair? If yes, what?

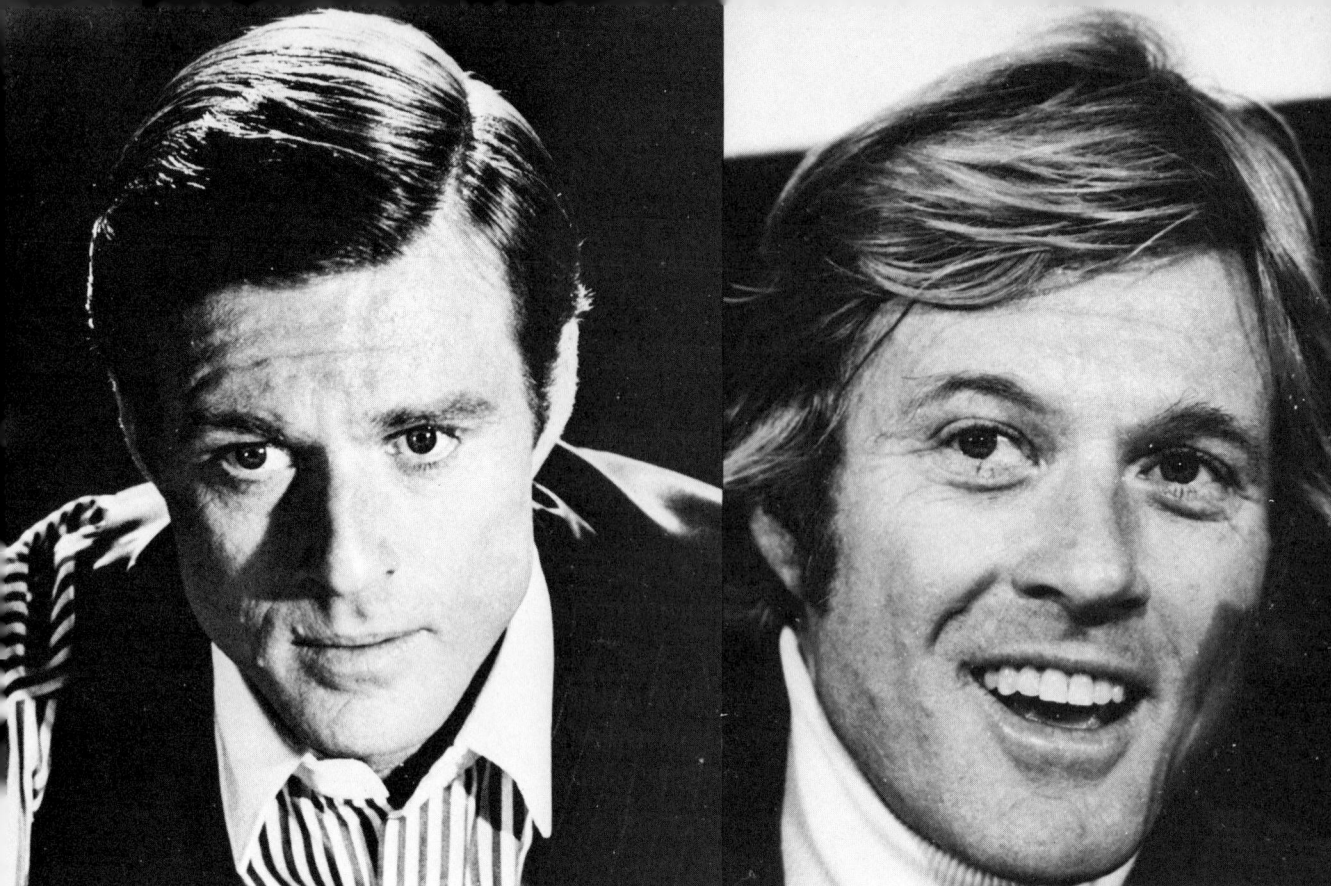

One haircut should give you at least two different looks. In The Great Gatsby, Redford's side-parted style was worn smooth, slick, and sophisticated. The look is easy to achieve with short-to-medium-length hair, using either a gel or an oily hair groomer. Apply the product through your damp hair with your fingers. Then comb neatly into place. A good formal business look. It can be tousled, as at right, for a casual look.

men—you will find out that your hair can do things you never imagined. Do you have thin or medium hair but wish your hair could look as thick as Sylvester Stallone's or John Travolta's? There's a strong possibility that it can.

This isn't merely a pep talk. Like most men, you probably have not thought a great deal about your hair. Unfortunately, you may have tried every barber on the block and every hair product, only to give up in the end and settle for a merely tolerable haircut. That's easy to understand.

But you have options you may not have considered. It could be simply a matter of changing your part to flatter the shape of your face, abandoning the blow-drying to let your natural wave emerge, or enhancing your hair color. You could add facial hair with a beard or moustache or permanent your hair to add lift and wave.

Combing, cutting, coloring, and shaping . . . all have the potential to make you look better.

The point: Within the range of your particular hair's abilities, you have many options for improving your looks.

Negative Thinking

There are a lot of people out there who will tell you that thinking about your hair is somehow unmanly. They will tell you to shampoo with whatever is in the shower—"It's all the same." They'll say you only need a haircut when your hair starts to brush the back of your shirt collar. They'll tell you it doesn't matter who cuts your hair and how. Hey, real men don't use conditioners on their hair, right?

Not true!

As you may already have discovered through exercise, relaxation techniques, motivational courses, or fine clothing, taking care of yourself is the only way to become the best man you can be. Attending to your hair is not a sign of unmanliness. It shows that you are out to become the best—and the best-looking—person you can be.

Positive Thinking

You probably don't need radical changes. Sometimes the simplest changes can create the most dramatic results. Changing a part from right to left can give the top of your hair more body automatically (the hair will be combed in the opposite direction to which it has been trained, so it will stand away from the scalp and look higher). Part-

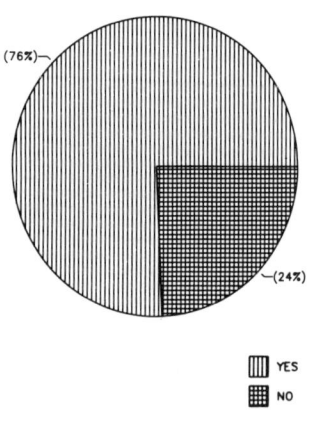

(76%)

(24%)

▥ YES
▦ NO

ing your hair higher or lower on your head can make your face look rounder, squarer, longer, thinner—whatever most benefits your looks. If you have a beard or moustache, it may just need the barest trimming to improve the shape of your face.

Even hair coloring, the last of men's taboos concerning hair, doesn't have to be radical. A discreet lightening or darkening of your hair can draw attention to your face in ways that will astonish you and delight the people who know you. They may not even know what has been changed, only that you look terrific.

No Complications

Men look better if they keep their haircuts simple. I like uncomplicated, easy-care cuts. With the right hairstyle you can let your hair dry naturally and comb it into place. Even if you need a routine to get the look you want, the routine shouldn't take more than ten minutes.

The David Frost Routine

An example of an easy routine that produces many benefits is the one I devised for David Frost, the television personality. I worked on David's hair for a week when he was hosting "Good Morning America." He has very fine hair. (Fine hair is narrow hair. If thick hair is the equivalent of rope, fine hair is like thread.)

David needs a routine to look his best. I used a blow dryer and a flat natural bristle brush (like a Mason & Pearson brush) to separate the fine hair strands while blow-drying. But, and this is important, even *before* drying, while the hair was damp, I sprayed on a setting lotion (such as Flex Set or Pantene Set). I sprayed the damp hair because setting lotion sticks to the damp strand and coats it more evenly than when dry. The fine glaze coating thickens the hair without any stickiness, partially because it blends with the water on the hair. Then I proceeded to blow-dry the hair, lifting it upward off the scalp.

The result: His hair actually looked thick and full. And the routine took all of ten minutes!

Synchronizing Your Hair and Personality

We all know people who look ill-fitted to their personalities. Why? It's often their hair. They could learn a few things from the people who work in front of cameras for a living.

For example, John Stossel is a consumer reporter for ABC Television. He is in his late thirties and has an extremely handsome face. He could probably make it in modeling if he weren't more interested in being a reporter for a major television network. When I first met John he looked very young and preppy. That, believe it or not, was the problem! As a consumer reporter, he wanted to project a more mature, believable image. His neat, perfectly groomed hair was standing in the way.

On my advice, John grew his hair longer, letting it touch his collar in back. That worked. With his longer hair, he looked more rugged, not so groomed. Before, he looked as if he might have spent hours on his hair every day. With longer hair, roughed up a bit, he became more powerful and authoritative on camera.

Hair can be out of sync with your facial structure and body shape, too, as was the case with Allen the singer. Another example from my client roster is Joel Siegel, entertainment reporter for ABC.

When I first met Joel, he was beginning a complete makeover of himself. At the time he was a bit portly, with lots of unruly hair, a huge moustache, and glasses. In truth, he looked like Gene Shalit.

Joel was losing weight but not fast enough. Since he wanted to look thinner, I gave him a haircut to help him speed up the "thinning" process. I cut his hair short on the sides and back, with more hair on top—no part, just tousled to add height. The short sides and fuller top slimmed his face. His hair became squarer, less round, which is a "thinner" shape. I also trimmed his moustache so that you could see his upper lip, because the bushy version makes a man's cheeks look fatter. He traded his glasses in for contacts.

The result: Joel was so encouraged by his new look that he stuck to his diet and trimmed down fast. His haircut gave him a whole new attitude. He looks and feels terrific.

A new look can do the same for you. It's easy to make a big difference in your appearance through uncomplicated and often downright simple hair styling techniques. I'm going to show you . . .

- *How to get the look you want;*
- *How to bring out your face's strengths;*
- *How to minimize any features you don't like;*
- *How to make your hair shiny, manageable, sexy;*
- *How to get your hair in sync with your life, your image, your personality;*
- *How to use moustaches and beards to further compliment your look.*

In the pages ahead, you'll find out that *you* can have great-looking hair, no matter what kind of hair you have now.

2.

HOW TO LOOK AT YOUR FACE

Analyzing Your Face:
The First Step to
a Great Haircut

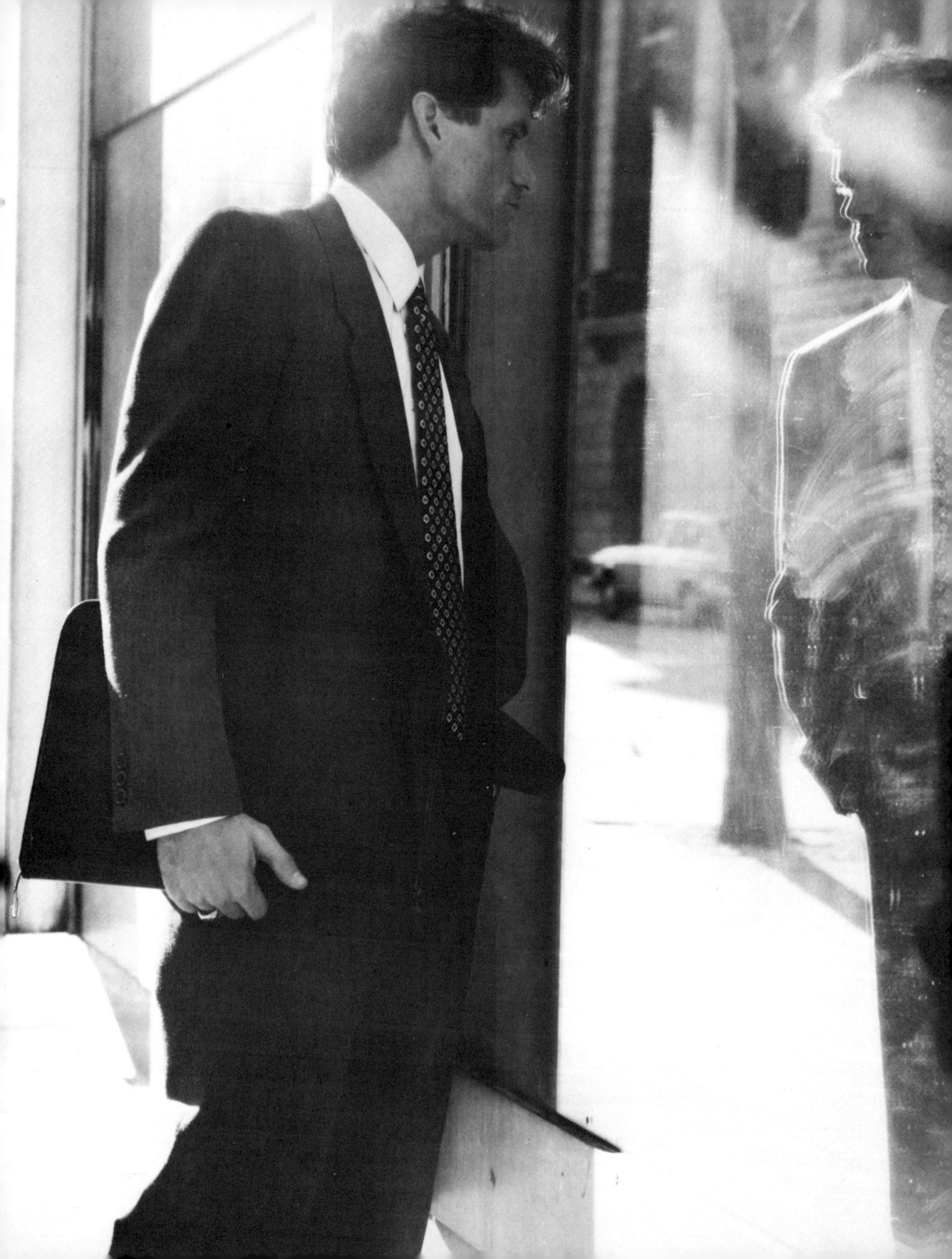

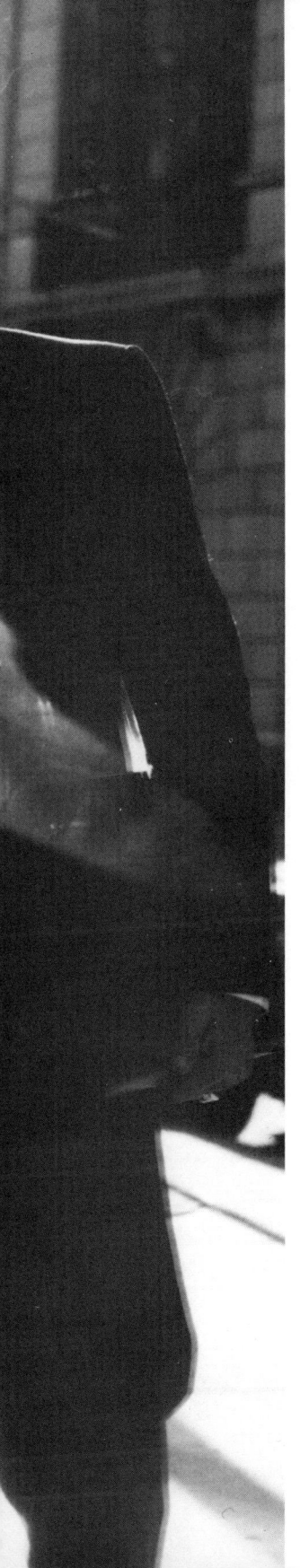

A Profitable Partnership: Your Face and Your Hair

To make the most of your hair, first you have to study and get to know your face. Why? Because your most successful hairstyle will be the one that works the best with your unique facial structure and features. You want your haircut to play up your most attractive points, play down your weaknesses.

I want you to look at your face as though you've never seen it before. I want you to analyze it as objectively as a portrait artist, breaking it down into proportions, outstanding features, shape, and bone structure.

Then we'll consider how you feel about your face:

- *What you like about it*
- *What gives it personality and character*
- *How to use it to project power, authority, love, friendliness*

I know you look at your face all the time—when you're shaving, brushing your teeth, combing your hair. You're probably quick to notice a patch of razor burn or a blemish. But if you are like most men, you take the basic structure of your face for granted.

I want you to take your face apart. Look at how each feature relates to your face as a whole and to your other features. Do this as objectively as you can, much the way you examine your body (if you work out) to check on the growing definition of

31

your stomach muscles or biceps, or in the way you buy a new suit, standing in front of a mirror checking the fit to see if your shoulders look broad and your waist nipped in.

You're going to discover the great things in your face: the features you can show off and feel terrific about, the places where your hairstyle can really help you balance proportions, add interest, or subtly camouflage features you'd rather keep in the background.

All it takes is a little homework, spending some time alone with yourself. Do it on a Sunday morning when the day is yours or on an evening after work, when you can play some soft music, mix a drink and, most important, *relax.*

When you're ready, go into the bathroom, where there is surely a mirror and good lighting and where you do most of your grooming. You'll need a second mirror, too, one you can hold. Then take off your shirt, so you can see your neck and shoulders clearly.

Now, wet your hair and slick it straight back so that it is flat against your head and behind your ears. (You want to make it seem to disappear.) You should now be able to see the true shape of your face and head.

The Basic Shapes

Look first at the shape of your face as a whole. With your hair slicked back, you should be able to see the outline of your face clearly. It will fit in roughly with the five basic shapes that follow, but bear in mind that nobody has a face that fits into an exact mold.

Hint: If you have trouble deciding on your basic shape, look straight into the mirror. Then outline your face on the mirror with a bar of soap. This will help you pinpoint your face-shape category.

The Round Face

The widest part of a round face is *straight across the cheekbones, from ear to ear.* The face is proportionately shorter than most; it appears almost as wide as it is long. (Ernest Borgnine, John Denver, and Dom DeLuise have round faces.)

Here's how your hair can work best with a round face.

- It can make your face look longer—with a beard or longer hair behind the ears.
- It can shape and define your chin—with the same technique, a beard and longer hair in back.
- It can add height to the top of your head—with a part closer to the center of the head or a tousle on the forehead. This breaks the round expanse of forehead.

The Square Face

Square faces are *equally wide at the jawbone and the forehead.* The key here is working with that wide jawbone either to dramatize it (like Dick Tracy or Superman) or play it down. *You* decide which way to go. (Phil Donahue and Mikhail Baryshnikov are real-life square faces.)

The Triangular Face

The triangular face is *wider at the jaw than at the forehead.* In this case you will probably want to balance the wide jaw by expanding the forehead.

Widen the top of your face by wearing your hair

- With a part near the side of the forehead,

drawing the eye away from the center of the face.

- In a style that adds fullness at the temples.

The Heart-Shaped Face

This shape is *wider at the forehead than at the jawline*. Often there is a pointed chin. (Jesse Jackson and Jimmy Connors come to mind.)

Your hair can help

- Deemphasize your forehead—by wearing an off-center part or a tousle on your forehead.
- Strengthen your jaw—by wearing hair longer behind the ears.

The Oblong Face

This face is *much longer than it is wide*. (Remember Prince Charles, Basil Rathbone, and David Hartman.) It is a very aristocratic look if handled well.

Use your hair

- To add width and extra fullness at the sides.
- To widen your forehead—with a part low on the side of the forehead.

The Oval Face

With this shape, *the cheekbone area is slightly wider than the forehead or jawline* and slightly above the center of the face.

If this is your face shape, you are lucky; you can wear almost any hairstyle. Choose one that brings out your best features.

A Question of Length

**Short hair is two inches long or shorter.
Medium hair is two to four inches long.
Long hair is four inches and longer.**

Face Proportions

Next, I want you to look into the mirror and mentally divide your face into three sections.

- Section One encompasses your forehead, from your hairline to the top of your eyebrows. (If your hairline is receding, go right up there. If you are bald, go to the top of your head.)
- Section Two covers the area from your eyebrows to the base of your nose.
- Section Three is the area from the base of your nose to the end of your chin.

The classic Greek ideal was a face in which these three areas were equal in size, but very few men have these proportions. This is where you can put your hairstyle to work for you—to create a better *balance* in your face.

Hint: Think highlight potential. When analyzing your facial features, ask yourself if you want to accent, or highlight, a special feature. Draw attention to your good points.

Keep highlight potential in mind. It's an important key to making your face look its best.

Section One: Your Forehead

Look straight into the mirror and concentrate on your forehead area.

- First look at the horizontal length to see if you have a wide or narrow forehead.
- Then look at the vertical length to see if your forehead is high or low.
- Determine if this is the largest of the three sections of your face.
- Look at the relationship of your forehead to

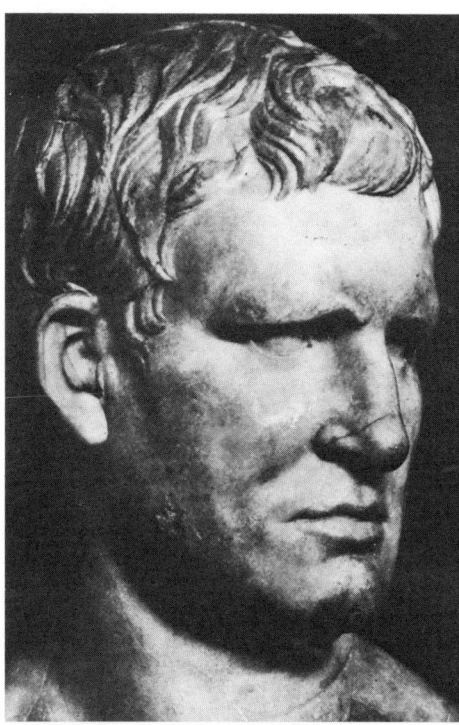

Today's good looks are based on proportions seen as ideal in ancient Greek culture.

WHAT DO YOU LIKE ABOUT YOUR FACE?

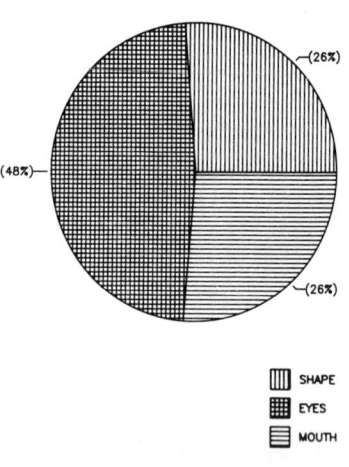

(26%)

(48%)

(26%)

	SHAPE
	EYES
	MOUTH

WHAT DO YOU DISLIKE ABOUT YOUR FACE?

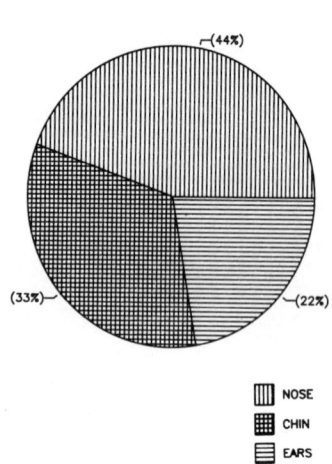

(44%)

(33%)

(22%)

	NOSE
	CHIN
	EARS

your hairline. If your hairline is high and receding, it will lengthen your face. If it is low, it will visually shorten your face.

Hint: Part hair strategically. One of the key decisions you will have to make when planning your haircut is where to place your part, if you want a part at all. Where you part your hair is an important device for narrowing or widening your entire face. It's an instant eye-catcher, an important diversionary tactic to draw the eye toward or away from a feature.

The closer your part is to the center of your face, the *narrower* your entire face will appear, specifically your forehead. The farther away from the center, the *wider.*

Your hair can help bring your forehead into balance with the rest of your face. It can create an illusion of height with more volume on top of the head. It can cover a high or receding hairline with a tousle falling onto the forehead. And, with clever placement of the part, it can create either an illusion of a wider or narrower expanse.

Section Two: Your Eyebrows, Eyes, Nose, Cheekbones, and Ears

The middle section of your face is full of highlight potential. First, consider your eyebrows.

Thick, dark eyebrows are a great asset. They frame the eyes, add strength and expressiveness to the face. Tom Selleck's bushy eyebrows are a dramatic focal point and counterbalance his famous moustache. If your eyebrows are very bushy and seem to overpower your face, you might consider growing a moustache like Tom's to balance them.

Thin, wispy eyebrows—like Fred Astaire's—can

Your Face
Analyze Your Features

Hairline
Show it off if it's clearcut, strong, or you just like it. Play it down if it's sparse, weak, or unflattering.

Forehead
Wide or narrow? High or low? Where you part your hair can do much to balance the proportions of your hair to your face and body.

Eyebrows
Thick and bushy or thin and wispy? Your eyebrows give expression to your face and draw attention to your eyes.

Eyes
They show your star quality and communicate your feelings more than any other feature.

Nose
It gives your face character. Noses that are too large or small are balanced with the right hair proportions.

Mouth
What does it express? Sensuous or circumspect? A moustache or beard could give you the qualities you desire.

Chin/Jaw
You can make it a positive feature. Knowing your facial structure is the key to deciding on the right hair length to strengthen your chin.

be colored to play them up. Or better yet, focus on another feature, your eyes.

Your eyes. The eyes are your—everyone's—single most important facial feature. More than anything else about your looks, they express your personality and emotions. Your eyes are full of highlight potential. Notice how intense their color is, how far apart they are spaced (according to the classic ideal, the space between your eyes should be the length of one eye), the size in relation to the rest of your face.

You can call attention to your eyes with a tousle of hair on the forehead. A low side-part (near the temples) will tend to widen close-set eyes. Hair two inches short on the sides of the head and sideburns trimmed to cheekbone height or above will open up the face and highlight your eyes.

Your nose. Noses come in as many configurations as fingerprints. You should not be concerned with the shape of your nose as much as with its size in relationship to your other features. Then consider the subjective factor—whether you like your nose and want to play it up or would rather distract attention from it.

If your nose is very large and overpowering, or if for some reason you dislike it, you can balance the midsection of your face by wearing longer hair in the back, showing below the ears. If your face is too dominated by your nose in profile, you can wear more hair on top of your head to balance side proportions.

If you have a small nose, you can make it more imposing with a shorter haircut.

Your cheekbones. Cheekbones give your face planes, depths, curves—in other words, character.

High cheekbones give added impact to the eyes and more definition and drama to the face. They are most noticeable on people with slimmer faces.

If you see rounded contours in the mirror instead of planes, take heart. You can create an illusion of cheekbones by shaving your sideburns so they stop at the center of the actual cheekbone. (More about this later.)

Your ears. The last features I want you to analyze in the middle portion of your face are not, strictly speaking, facial features at all. However, your ears *can* determine what haircut works for you.

If your ears are too big or stick out, you know it already. Stick with a haircut that grazes the ears, partially covering them. Another option is to grow hair fuller behind your ears to camouflage their proportion and structure.

If you think your ears look great, no matter how large or small they are, count them as an asset and show them off. The point is to bring your ears in sync with the rest of your face.

Hint: Bland is boring. I've seen many harmonious faces that look dull and uninteresting because they have no emphasis, no facial feature that stands out.

Accenting a strong facial feature is exciting. Don't think only of covering up a standout feature. That may be the very thing that makes your face unique and memorable.

Section Three: Your Lips, Chin, and Jaw

Your lips. A good smile is important. You want to make the most of yours. Sensuous lips can be another plus. If your mouth is low-key or you have very thin lips, think about growing a moustache.

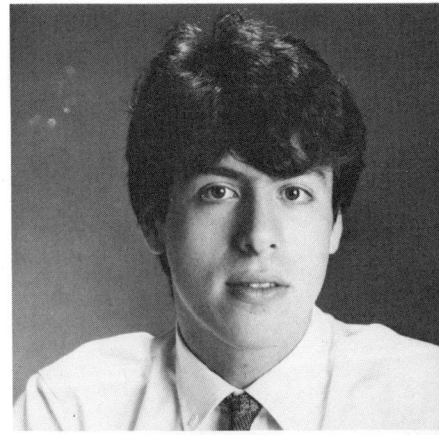

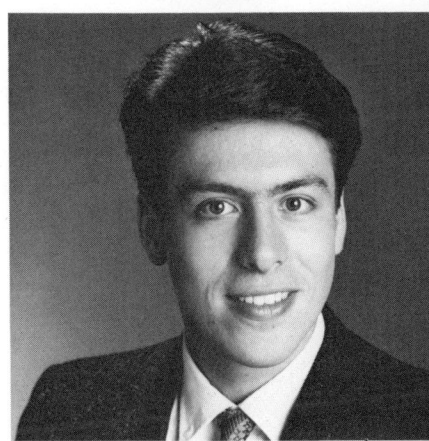

Jairo has thick, wavy, dark hair. It was out of shape and hung in his face. The length wasn't as much of a problem as the shape. Removing the hair on the sides of his head opened up his eye and cheek area, making his eyes appear larger. I gave him a side-part and used an oily groomer to get the hair up and off his face. The result: a more professional-looking Jairo.

A different hairstyle really can't do much to minimize or highlight your mouth, but moustaches certainly can. For example, a moustache will fill in the gap over a thin lip, adding a much-needed anchor to the face. It will play up your teeth and dramatize your smile. (Stacy Keach balances his face with a moustache.)

Your chin and jaw. Your chin and jaw are at the bottom of your face, but they're among your top facial features. Look to see what shape your jaw gives to the general contour of your face. The line of your chin and jaw, whether decidedly square, pointed, or rounded, largely determines your face shape.

Your haircut can help fill in the lower portion of your face if you have a pointed or small chin. For this, the style you wear should have visible hair behind the ears to widen the lower part of your face.

A prominent square jaw calls for shorter hair. (But men's hair is often cut too short to have any impact on the lower region of the face.)

Beards can work miracles in the jaw area. If you have a heart-shaped face (wide forehead, small jaw and chin) and feel that your face looks weak because of it, growing the proper beard will give your jaw a squarer, stronger shape.

Your Profile

It's easy for you and for a hair stylist to concentrate on the face, which is what you see when you look straight on in the mirror, and neglect the profile and back of the head. But out there in the world people see you from all angles, profile included. So while you are at the mirror, let's get a view of you from the side.

I hope you are enjoying this process of self-discovery, but I know there is an outside chance that you are feeling embarrassed at looking at yourself so carefully. Don't worry. That's a natural reaction. Accept the fact that you may feel self-conscious. It isn't every day that you take a real look at yourself. Take time to get to know every feature on your face. Each new insight will bring you a step closer to a better hairstyle.

Turn to the side and lift your chin. Using the hand mirror to see your reflection in the larger mirror, look at your hairline; scan down your forehead, over your eyebrows, your nose, lips, and chin. Look once more, taking in your profile as a whole.

Ideally, your forehead and chin should be parallel. However, your chin may protrude or recede from the plane formed by your forehead. If it protrudes, chances are it looks strong. No problem. But a receding chin can look weak, and if this bothers you, here's where your hair can do a balancing act.

- Longer hair at the sides of the head (covering all but the lower half inch of the ear) will make the chin look wider.
- At the same time, hair in back of the ear should be grown longer and thicker to fill in the lower third of the face.
- Hair on the back of the head should be worn collar length, to balance the receding chin in profile.

The Shape of Your Head

Still using your hand mirror and staying in profile, look at the shape of your head from your hairline to the base of your neck. Is the curve of your head smooth, or do you have a flat top at your crown? If you have such a flat area—and most men do—your hair volume can be adjusted to compensate.

The Back of Your Head

The back of your head is a hidden asset. People see you going as well as coming.

Hold your hand mirror so you can see a rear view of your head. With your free hand, push the hair back there up and off your neck.

Proportion is everything when it comes to styling the hair on the back of your head. We're talking about the relationship of your head to your neck and shoulders. If your neck is either short and wide or long and thin, you can improve the proportion with your hairstyle.

A short wide neck can be slimmed down
- By hair cut in a V or U shape in back.
- By wearing hair higher on top of the head.

A long thin neck gets the illusion of width
- By wearing slightly longer hair, a half inch below your shirt collar.

Your Strong Points

Now that you're really familiar with your face, it's time to make some judgments about what you do and don't like about it. Before drying your hair, get a pen and paper and come back to the mirror. I want you to make a list of your facial best bets, the ones you want your hair to play up.

These can be any part of your face or upper body that you feel brightens up your image. Here are some clues to help you.

- **Bone structure.** The older you get, the more your face's bone structure shows, assuming you have stayed in shape. A good, sharply defined bone structure is what usually makes handsome men handsome. For example, brow bones that protrude can draw attention to your eyes and make them look strong. Protruding cheekbones or a thick jaw also adds strength to your face. If your face doesn't have a strong bone structure, I'll show you how to

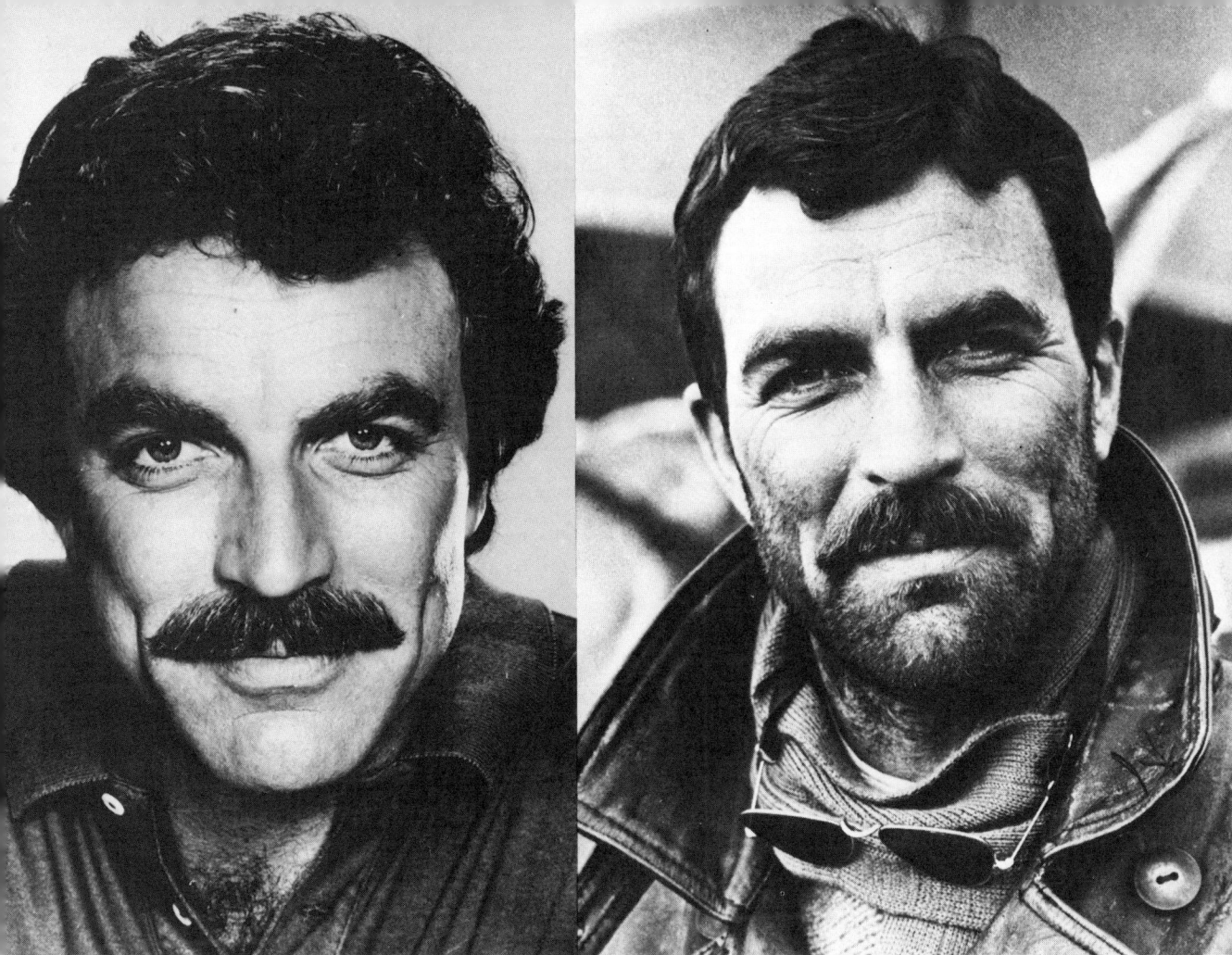

create the effect of good bones with the right hairstyling.

- **Eyes.** I believe everyone's eyes are a strong point. Note the color, size, and expressiveness of yours. Even if you don't particularly care for your eyes, the right hairstyle can make them a plus. I'll show you how!

- **Hairline.** If you have a good, defined hairline like Ronald Reagan, write it down by all means. You need a haircut that shows it off.

Whatever features you choose to put on your list can be accentuated and complemented with your hair. What's important here is to decide now,

Tom's hair changes roles easily.

Medium-length wavy hair gives Tom Selleck a softer, sexy look. His classic moustache balances his thick eyebrows. The strict, short military hair played against a rugged beard gives Tom the rough and ready magnetism for his aviator role. Two totally different looks, both exuding sex appeal.

43

subjectively what you like about your face. Then we'll work toward a hairstyle that brings out these points, one that makes you feel great about yourself.

What to Play Down

Note the features you would like to minimize in your face. We've mentioned several possibilities, such as a receding hairline, receding chin, large or small nose, large forehead, wispy eyebrows, a thin upper lip, a thin neck.

Don't take these flaws too seriously. As I have said before, you can live easily with features you don't like by adopting the right hairstyle and/or facial hair.

Look at how your face has changed in the past five, ten, or twenty years. Many men subconsciously cling to an outdated image of their face as it looked in their school yearbooks. Don't think that all change in your face is undesirable. With age comes character, one of the most attractive qualities you can possess.

You should also be aware of how your face looks when you use it—when you talk, laugh, frown, grimace. Act into the mirror. Look happy, pensive, sad, bitter, even crazy! Stretch your face to its emotional and physical limits. Have fun. Push your hair back with your fingers and give yourself an intense stare.

Will this help you decide on a specific hairstyle for your face's features? Not yet. But it will increase your awareness of your face and the kind of hair that should go with it. Once you know your features and how they work, you are ready to make the most of what you have.

3.

HOW TO LOOK AT YOUR HAIR

Be Proud of Your Own Hair Qualities and Work with Them

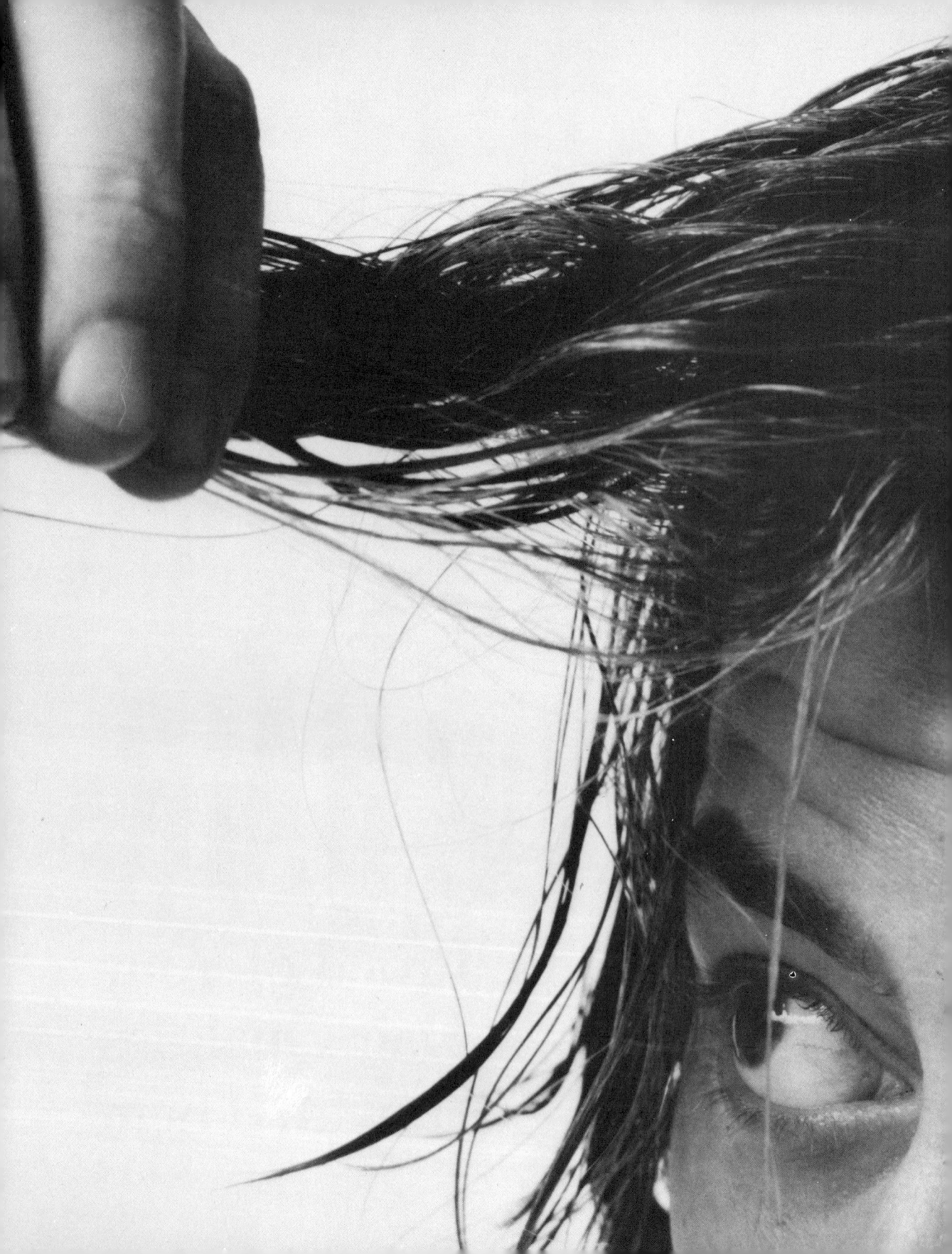

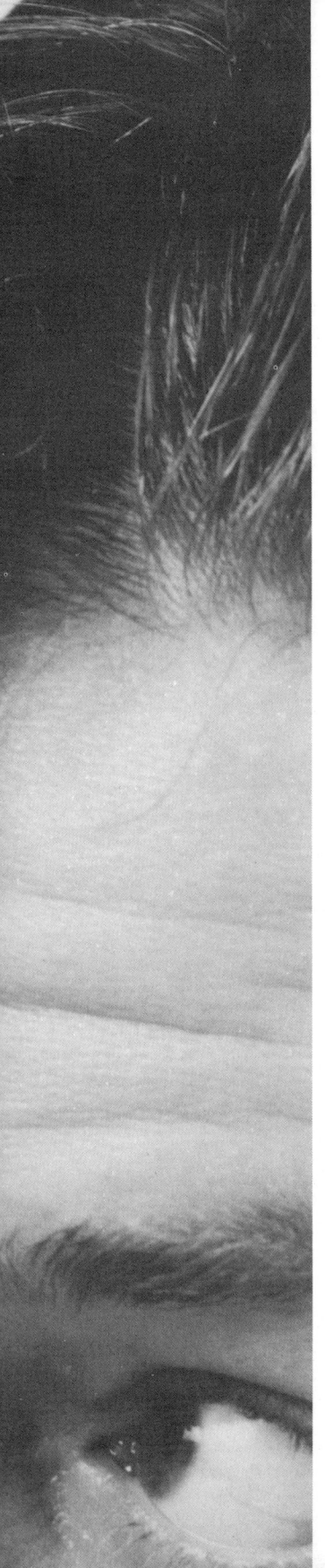

What a "Pro" Knows (about Your Hair)

You've spent hours shampooing, drying, combing, brushing, and fussing with your hair, but do you really know it? I'm going to show you how to look at your hair with the objectivity of a professional hair stylist—to see it in a new way.

Everything about your hair is special—its color, its shine, the direction it grows in naturally on your head, its texture, its thickness. You may have thick and dark hair or thin and lightly colored hair, as many men do. Whatever the case, your particular head of hair has too many colors, textures, and other variables to be duplicated.

There are some things you may not yet know about your hair. And you can learn about them only if you spend time analyzing your hair the way I would if you were my client (and, through this book, you are). So, if you discovered something new about your features when looking at your face, this chapter should really start you on the fast track toward a great hairstyle.

Hair: The Basics

I've said your hair is unique. It is. But all hair is alike in some basic ways. For example, all hair is dead. (If hair were alive like other parts of your body, would you want to get it cut?)

Each strand (or shaft) of hair on your head is

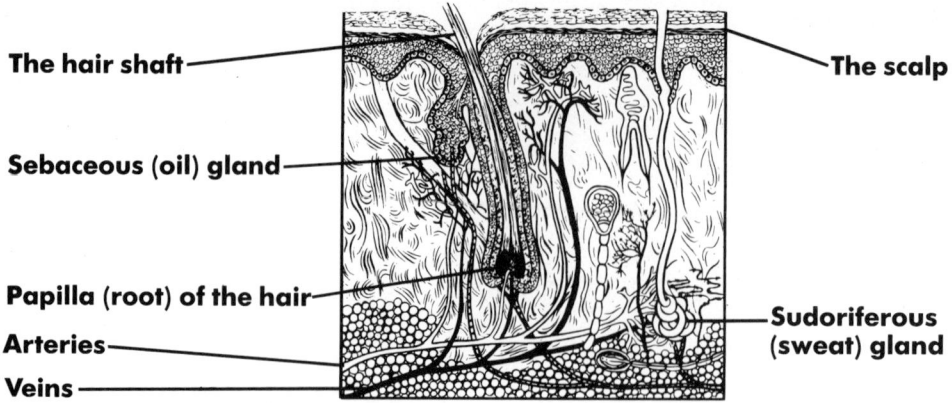

The hair shaft

The scalp

Sebaceous (oil) gland

Papilla (root) of the hair

Arteries

Veins

Sudoriferous (sweat) gland

made of a type of protein called keratin. Hair shafts are produced by follicles in your scalp and are pushed up like spring grass to where we can see them.

At first glance at a head of hair, you would think the hair shafts are perfectly round, a kind of soft wire, but they're not. There is an exterior cuticle protecting an inner cortex. If you looked under a microscope, you would see that the cuticle looks like overlapping layers of fish scales.

The cortex contains chemicals that determine the formation of your hair (straight, wavy, curly, or a combination of these), depending on the way these chemicals are bonded together. The cortex also contains the pigment granules, or melanin, that dictate the color of your hair. If these granules are medium in size and distributed evenly throughout the shaft, you will be the proud owner of red hair. Lots of large granules distributed unevenly result in brown hair shafts; fewer, smaller granules make the blond shades.

So much for the basic theme. Now for the variations.

Hair Characteristics

As a "pro," I look at four separate but equally important characteristics of your hair: *texture, con-*

dition, *amount of hair on your head, and formation* (*curly, straight, etc.*). Within each of these four categories are several possibilities.

It's important to treat each characteristic separately, to make it the best it can be, and to minimize any weak spots. You'll want to get all four properties working together the best they can to enhance your looks.

Texture

Say you have just come to me for a haircut. First, I'd want to check the texture of your hair. This will tell me how well your hair will hold a shape.

As a general rule, hair texture is categorized by the *width* of the strand;

- Fine hair has the least width.
- Medium is a bit thicker.
- Coarse is thickest in width and best able to hold a shape.

But please note: Your hair's texture can vary in different places on your head. You may have coarse sideburn hair around your ears and into the nape of your neck, while your top hair could be finer. Or you may be losing hair on top of your head, which is becoming coarse and wiry before it falls out, while the rest of your hair remains normal texture.

Hair texture can also vary from season to season. It can be coarser in summer and winter, due to sun-bleaching, heat, or wearing hats, than it is in the spring or fall.

If you have been blow-drying, chemical processing, or conditioning your hair, you can alter the natural texture. Go by the following test to discover the texture that your hair is now.

WHAT IS YOUR HAIR TEXTURE?

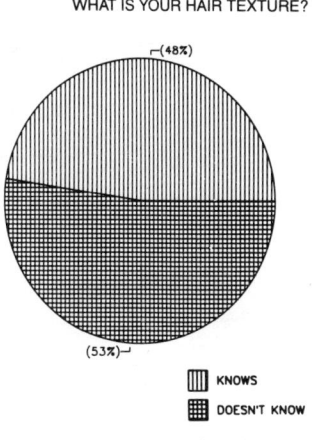

(48%)

(53%)

▥ KNOWS
▦ DOESN'T KNOW

Texture Test One

Check the descriptions in each box that apply to your hair. The box with the most checks will reveal your hair's basic texture. (If you want to keep your book intact, make a photocopy of this page and keep your own work sheet.)

Fine

( ) Your hair is soft.

( ) Your hair is flat in the morn-ing—it seems stuck to your head.

( ) You need to blow-dry your hair every day.

( ) You don't use conditioners on your hair be-cause they make it too soft.

( ) It is hard to keep your hair out of your face.

( ) You sometimes shampoo it twice a day.

Medium

( ) You can comb your hair in the morning, and it keeps its shape throughout the day.

( ) Blow-drying and drying naturally both give you a good look.

( ) Your hair looks good upon awakening.

( ) You skip using a creme rinse several times a week because you don't need it for manageability.

( ) You don't have to shampoo every morning. You sometimes only shampoo once every two or three days.

Coarse

( ) Your hair looks dull, even after shampooing.

( ) In the morning you can comb your hair into place without wetting it and have the style look right.

( ) You have to use conditioners on your hair, or it looks "wild" and/or dryed out.

( ) You can go for days without shampooing.

( ) Your hair feels rough.

( ) Your hair grows full instead of long.

Texture Test Two

This test can confirm the results of Texture Test One or, if you are still not sure of your hair's texture, help you discover it.

Here is how it works: Shampoo your hair, lathering only once and skipping any creme rinses or conditioners. (They tend to mask the hair's true texture.) Instead of vigorously drying your hair, blot out excess water with a towel and let it dry naturally. No combing. No brushing.

Now look.

- Fine hair will lie close to the head, with no "lift" off the scalp.
- You will notice some lift if you have medium-textured hair.
- Coarse hair will have a definite lift off the scalp and may look and feel dry, as if it really misses a creme rinse.

Texture Test Three

This test is more than a test for texture; it is also a way for you really to get to know your hair. It should be done soon after Texture Test Two for best results, when hair is naturally dry—no combing or brushing.

Here is how it works. Using both hands, fingers slightly open, start at your temples and run your fingers through your hair toward the crown of your head. While your hands move through your hair, ask yourself these questions:

- Is my hair easy to slide through?
  Imagine running your hands over a silk scarf. If your hair feels like silk, it's probably *fine.*
- Is there some resistance as my hands move through my hair?
  Sticking with the fabric example, this sensation would be more like a cotton T-shirt than a silk scarf. You probably have *medium*-textured hair.
- Is there a rough feeling to my hair; does it feel grainy?
  This would feel more like a nubby tweed than silk or cotton. If your hair feels this way, it is probably *coarse.*

Condition

If your hair is in great condition, you know it. It's smooth and shiny and does what you ask it to do. Your hair's overall shine and smoothness is a magnification of what's happening on the surface of your individual hair strands. You will remember that hair strands are covered with a cuticle made of "scales." When these scales lie on top of each other in a tight formation, they create a miniature mirror, reflecting light and giving your hair shine. Hair in poor condition is like a broken mirror. When the cuticle's scales are roughed up or broken off, hair becomes dull and weakened.

The cuticle's condition is partly determined by the scalp. The scalp produces an oily substance, sebum, which works its way onto hair shafts, coating the cuticle to give it sheen, smoothness, and flexibility. Since the hair you can see on your head is dead, this is the only nourishment it receives from the body.

Dry, normal, oily—what condition is your hair in? Find the description below that fits your hair best:

- **Dry.** When you wake up you can easily comb your hair into place. You don't like to shampoo every day, because if you do, your hair looks too fluffy. You like to use creme rinse and conditioners to tame your hair. Your scalp never feels oily.
- **Normal.** You could shampoo every day, but you don't have to. Your hair looks okay if you skip a day.
- **Oily.** You shampoo once a day, if not more. When you get out of bed in the morning, your hair lies flat on your head. You don't like to use creme rinses or conditioners because they leave your hair stringy.

Note: Your hair can fluctuate between two of the above categories. It may be normal most days, then move into an oily stage. Similarly, dry hair can become normal for a week or two before turning dry again. This is because the amount of oil produced by the scalp varies with such factors as stress, environment, diet, and hormonal fluctuations.

Hint: Very dry hair can sometimes swing into normal if you use a creme rinse every day. The buildup will fill in the rough, cracked cuticle.

● Oily hair can be shampooed once or twice a day. Cutting down on oils and fried foods in the diet can also help.

● Brushing the scalp stimulates oil production. Cut down or step up brushing according to your hair's condition.

● Many times your hair type will match your skin—for example, dry flaky skin accompanies dry hair; oily skin accompanies oily hair.

Amounts

You have noticed, I'm sure, that not all men have the same amount of hair on their heads—or on their bodies, for that matter. Whether your hair is coarse or fine, oily or dry, the amount you have depends on the number of hair shafts per square inch on your head. For now, forget about whether or not you're losing some of those shafts.

Let's label the amount of hair you have as *thin*, *medium*, or *thick*. As a general rule, brunettes have the thickest hair, blonds have less, and redheads the least (though many seem to have fountains of hair because it is usually coarse in texture). Here are two tests to determine the amount you have.

Magnified Hair Shaft

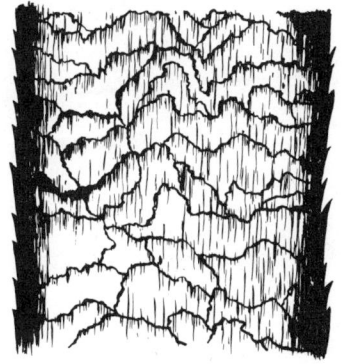

The cuticle is the outside layer of your hair shaft. As you can see in the magnified view of this hair shaft, the cuticle is actually made up of overlapping layers of cells, much like fish scales or tree bark. The flatter the scales lie, the smoother and shinier your hair. If the cuticle cells are roughed up or broken off, your hair will look dry and unshiny. Deep moisture conditioning can make the cuticle lie flatter; so can rinsing your hair with cool water.

The Wet Test

Wet your hair thoroughly (or do this test when you get out of the shower). Then check to see which of these descriptions describes your wet hair best:

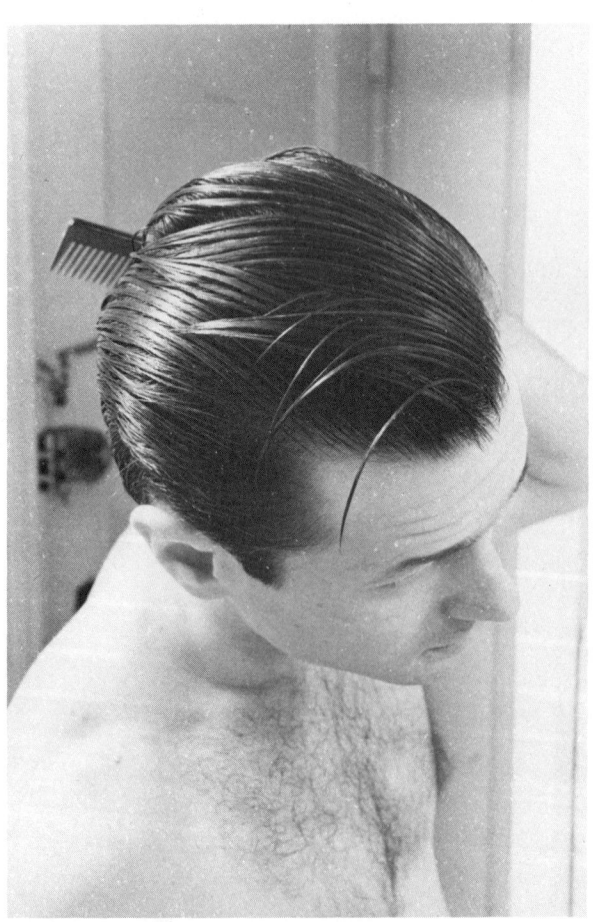

- *Thin.* You can easily and clearly see your scalp.
- *Medium.* You can barely see your scalp—it only shows in areas where your hair is thinning.
- *Thick.* You cannot see your scalp unless you part the hair and go looking.

- *Thin* hair dries quickly, in as little as a half hour in a room at comfortable temperature. You can usually dry thin hair in less than five minutes with a blow dryer.
- *Medium* hair will take a half hour to an hour to dry naturally, up to ten minutes when blown dry.
- *Thick* hair usually takes over an hour to dry naturally and up to fifteen minutes to dry with a blower.

The Dry Test

A simple rule of thumb when judging the amount of hair you have is that the longer your hair takes to dry, the thicker it is.

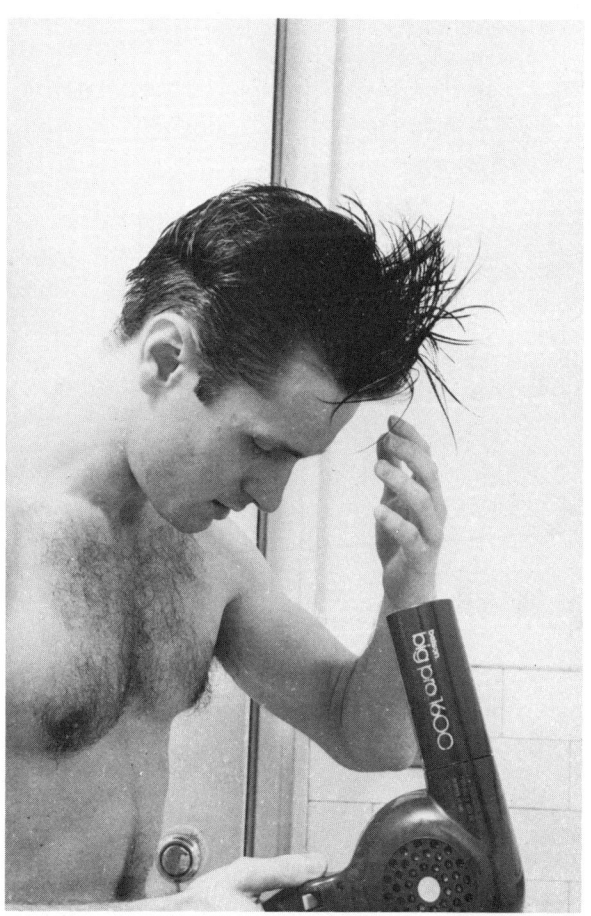

The Formation of Your Hair

A man's hair can take many forms. But most men's hair falls into three categories:

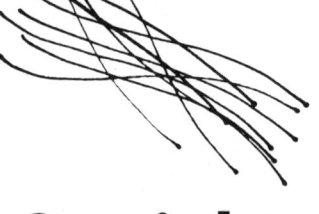 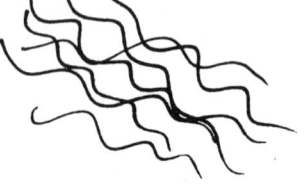 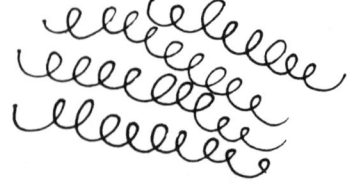

Straight   Wavy   Curly

As I mentioned before, these forms are the outcome of chemical bonds within the hair shafts. Each form of hair lends itself to certain general hair looks.

- Straight hair is better worn short to medium length.
- Wavy hair can be worn any length that suits your face.
- Curly hair will curl more when short. When longer, the weight will make it more wavy.

You may have several different kinds of hair on your head—curly in some places, kinky or wavy in others. Later we'll decide if you will want to work *with* these differing forms or if you'll want to make the hair appear the same all over. Bear in mind that you don't have to homogenize the different kinds of hair on your head. If handled properly, your hair can be naturally good-looking by using its different aspects to advantage.

Knowing your hair's formation will help guide you to the right cut.

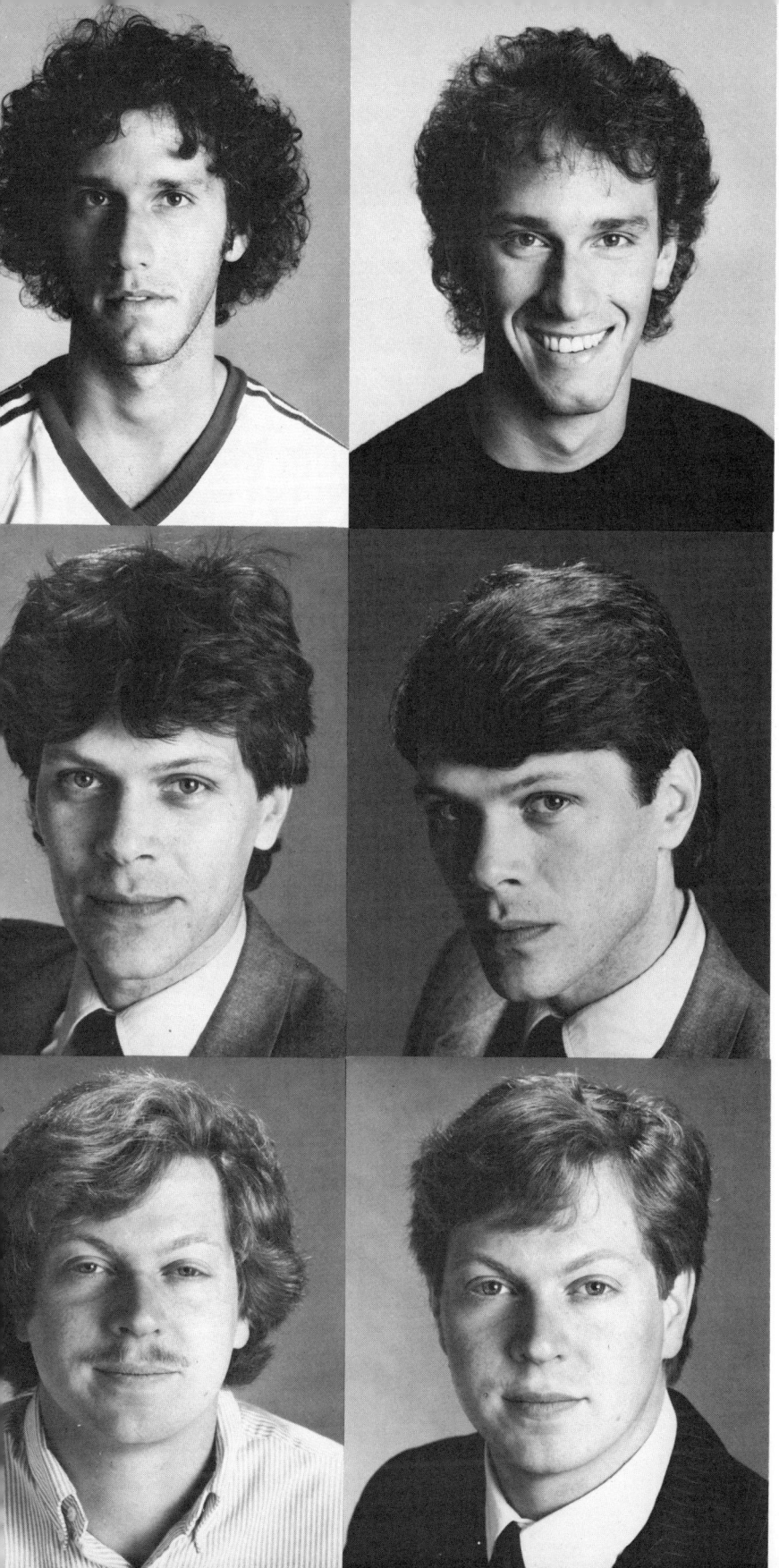

Fine

Fine-textured hair means the diameter of each hair is very small. Tony has fine, curly hair, which appears thicker than it actually is. The big round haircut does nothing to show off Tony's best facial features. The shorter, squarer cut makes his hair feel and act fuller. Again, the shorter hair on the sides widens his face and opens up the cheekbone and eye area. Fine hair needs daily shampooing, a finishing rinse, and a body-building groomer to look its best.

Medium

Medium-textured hair means that the diameter of the hair is neither too fat nor too thin. Gary has a thick amount of hair, a medium texture, and a slight wave. To balance Gary's long face, I removed the bulk from the top of his hair to eliminate a top-heavy look. By shortening the hair on the sides of his head, his face appeared wider and not quite so long. His medium-textured hair is easy to maintain. With regular haircuts and easy daily grooming, his hair looks great.

Coarse

Ken has coarse hair. This means each hair on his head is large in diameter and a bit rough-feeling. Coarse hair is often mistaken for thick hair because each individual hair takes up so much space. It needs deep-conditioning to control and add manageability. It holds a shape best in short to medium lengths. It should be shampooed every other day at most so as not to promote dryness. Use a creamy shampoo to add moisture. A dab of an oily groomer will help keep hair in place and add shine.

You've Got the Facts

You now know your face—what you want to show off, what you want to keep backstage. And you know your hair—its texture, condition, amount, and formation. This is what you have to work with, your raw material.

Now we're going to mold it into the look that's right for you. You have your tools, so let's make plans to bring out your best features, your hair's full potential.

4.

HOW TO FIND YOUR LOOK

It's Time to Let Your Haircut Reveal Who You Are *Now*

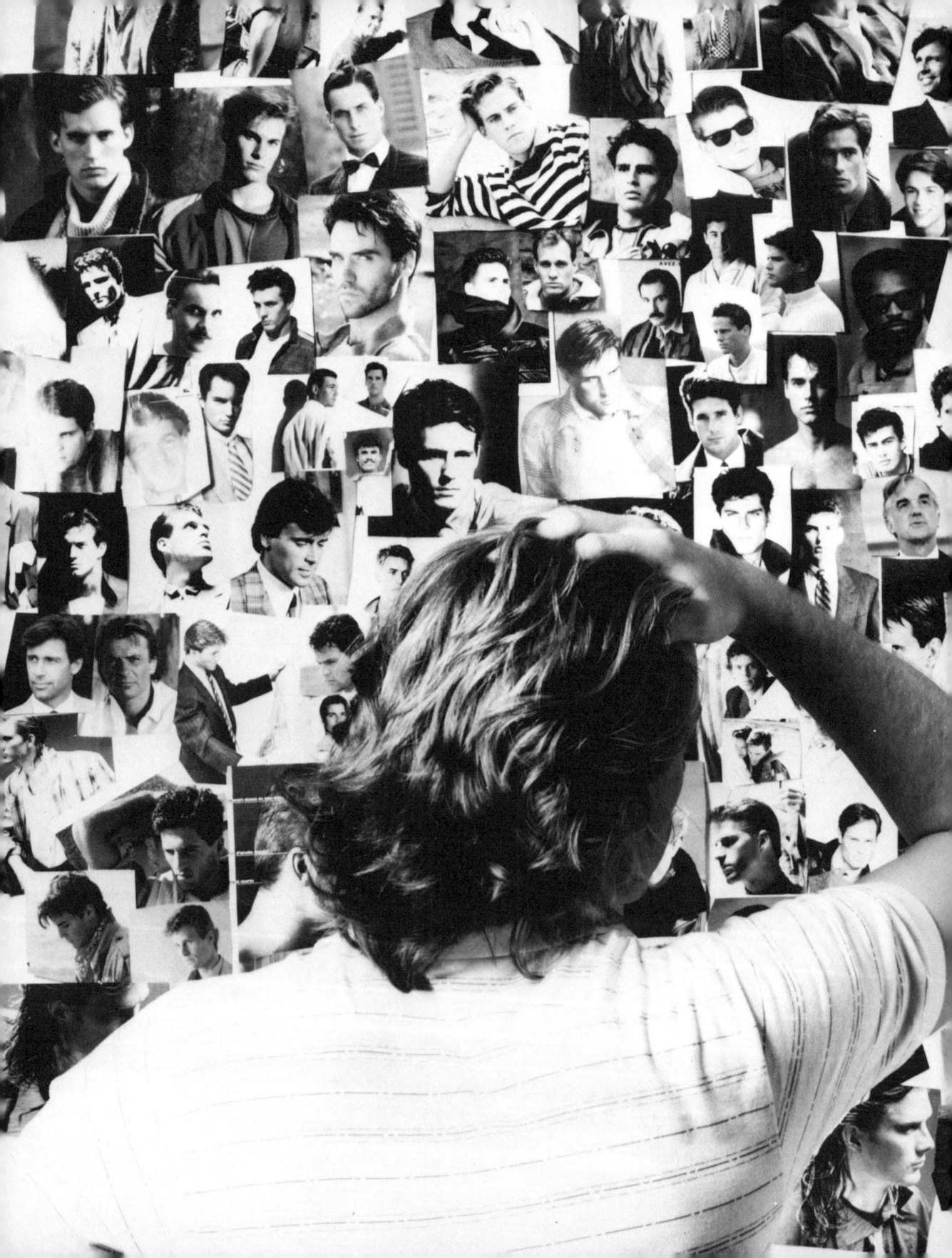

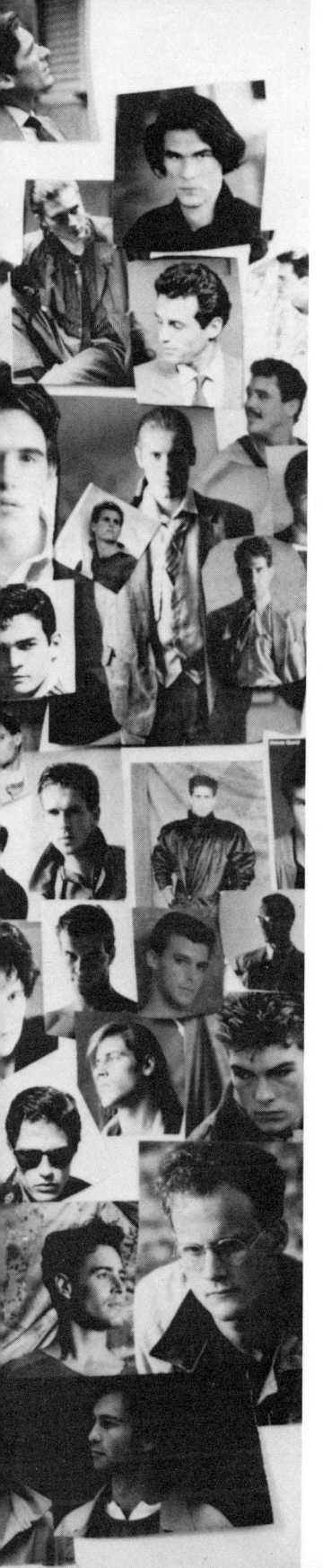

Knowledge Is Power

You are now armed with enough information about the basic potential of your hair and your face to put them to work for you.

This chapter is about taking charge of your looks, putting all your best facial features together with your particular hair and coming out with the best haircut for you. It should make the inner you feel comfortable. It should suit both your business image and your playtime.

Let's make it happen. Every haircut tells a story and you want yours to tell the world about *you*.

Getting Rid of a Stale Image

Part of keeping up with the changes in life is looking like the person you are at the moment, always striving to be the best version of you. But many men have left their look in the *past*.

It's important to face the fact that you do not have the same face that you had even a few years ago. Every year you gain a truer sense of yourself. It's time to show this in your looks.

You know about your strengths and limitations from the last chapters. Now let's go on to your life.

Think about your average day. You should be able to get dressed and ready for work effortlessly, knowing you look right for your job. Your hair should take you through the day, boosting your confidence and feeling of being in charge. If you are involved in sports or work out at a gym, you should not have to think about your hair. If you have a party or an elegant evening ahead, your hair should adapt to your change in wardrobe.

You can have it all: a cool, efficient hairstyle that looks controlled and confident on the job, hair that stays out of your way in athletics, and hair that looks elegant, with-it, and sexy at night.

Right now, think about the qualities you want your appearance to project.

Your Hair Can Give You a "Power Look"

Most of the time, you are going to be concerned about how your hair looks at work.

First of all, office hair should look like its owner is in control. For most men this means hair should be kept medium to short in length, because longer hair is easily disheveled.

It also means using a hair groomer if that's what it takes to keep your hair in place. Just a few years ago, television commercials were touting the dry look. Today it's okay to have a little shine in your hair. It shows you care enough to control it.

For examples of power hair, look to politics: Ronald Reagan's immaculately groomed style, Jesse Jackson's short, neat curls, Walter Mondale's silver sweep, and Gary Hart's controlled wave. Henry Kissinger's receding waves and Alexander Haig's modified military look also convey power and authority. Each man has a different kind of hair and face. Each has a "power look."

Note that hair on the sides and back of the head is usually cut shorter—three-quarters of an inch to two inches shorter than the hair on top of the

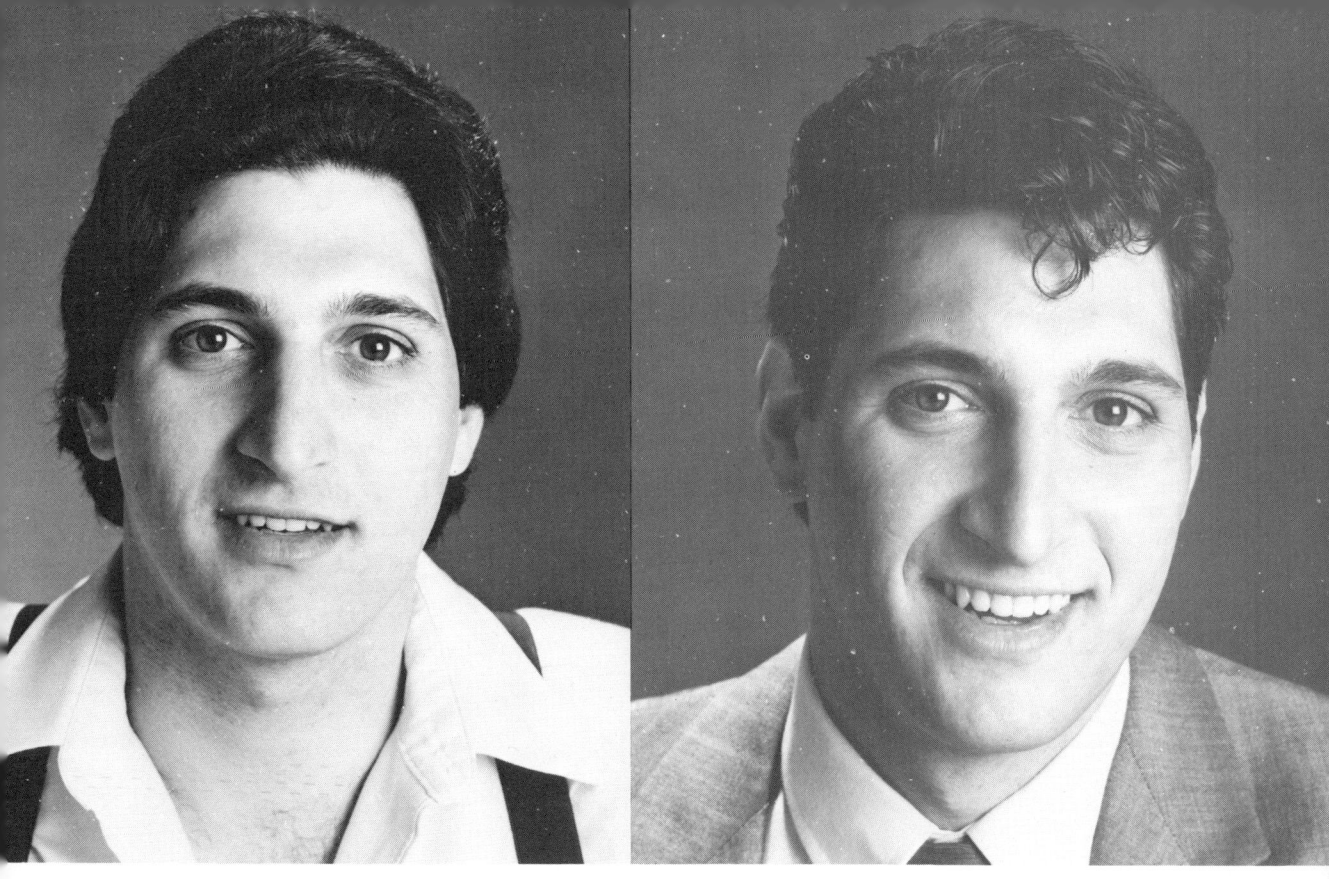

Steven

I cut Steven's hair shorter at the sides to expose his ears, which widens Section Two of his face, the eye/cheekbone area. His hair was then thinned slightly to add movement and texture. A hair groomer keeps the style soft. The tousle on his forehead highlights his beautiful eyes.

Steven wasn't using the potential of his thick, coarse hair.

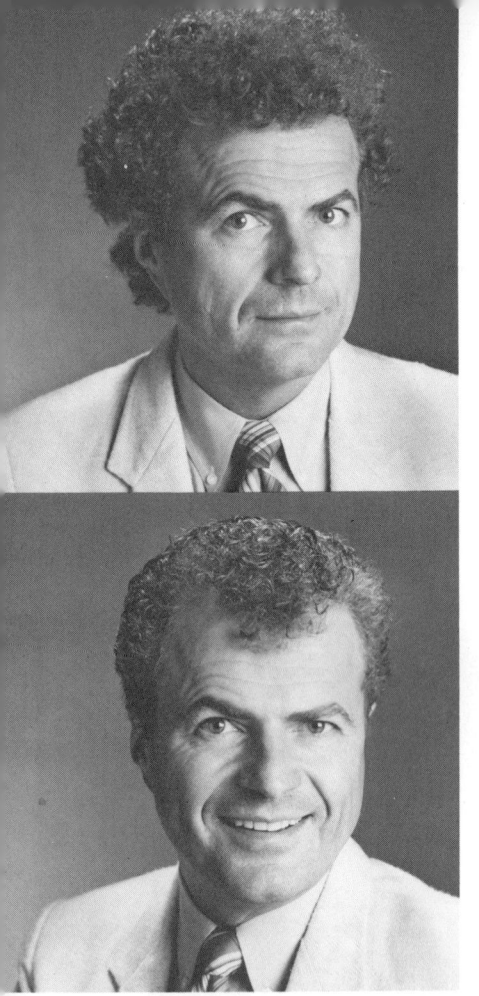

Marte has thick, blond, curly hair. The big bushy shape in his "before" photo detracts from his professional image. To give him a "power look," I thinned the hair to remove excess bulk. Then I cut his hair short on the sides to play up his eyes. The tousle on top minimizes his large forehead and also dramatizes his eyes. For easy maintenance, he shampoos every other day and uses an oily hair groomer to combat dryness.

head, which is kept proportionately longer (one and a half to four inches long). The more hair a man has, the longer he can grow his office hair, because thick hair will hold a neat shape.

The hair on the sides of the head should never completely cover the ears. That usually will be construed as saying you're hiding something. At the most, only the top third of the ears should be covered.

Long sideburns are out for the "power look." Keep them short and trimmed to cheekbone level or just above or below. They should be *no longer* than just under the cheekbone. Moustaches and facial hair also should be kept immaculate and beautifully trimmed, never flamboyant. (Jesse Jackson's Fu Manchu moustache was trimmed for the 1984 presidential campaign.)

How You Can Get the Sexy Look

What man doesn't want to look sexy and virile at some time of his life, if not every day? Ask a woman what turns her on in men's hair. You may be surprised at the answer. It's more the quality of a man's hair than the quantity. Shine, softness, touchability rate highest with the opposite sex.

• For sexy hair, your priority should be to get it in the best condition possible, so that it is sensual to the touch. That means clean, smelling good, feeling soft.

• Sexy hair is hair that moves. Leave off the heavy hair groomers and let your hair fall naturally. If a tousle falls a bit over your face, even better! It will call attention to your eyes.

• Nothing is less sexy than obviously artificial hair or hair that is too slicked down, controlled, unmovable.

- Rich color, sun streaks, and beautiful gray shading win points.

- Long hair can be very sexy if it is kept clean, healthy, and shaped—not too wild. The main concern with long hair is to keep it shiny and beautifully conditioned. Otherwise, it's a mess.

- Facial hair can give many men an instant macho look, especially if it masks a weak upper lip or a receding chin. But your facial hair should be touchable, never scratchy. Who wants to kiss a brush?

If your hair is nondescript and safe, it's not doing anything for your sex appeal. Consider a permanent wave to add body and movement, or coloring to enrich your natural shade. Think of adding healthy sun streaks. Most coloring products will also boost your hair by adding a new shine as a bonus.

While we're on the subject of sexy hair, let's get rid of some outdated notions of what is masculine and what is not. Today *any* hair can look masculine if it does the most for your facial features. Waving, coloring, growing your hair to your shoulders— don't rule *anything* out if it can help your looks.

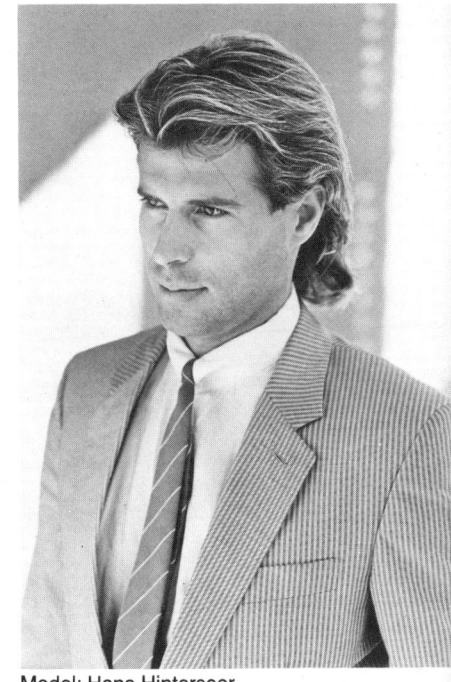

Model: Hans Hinterseer

Creative Hair—Do You Dare?

Some jobs allow a lot more leeway with a man's hairstyle. These are usually creative or teaching jobs, where you're also allowed more freedom of expression in your wardrobe. In fact, you may be expected to follow the latest trends, to be *au courant* with your hair as well as your clothes.

My advice is to enjoy yourself, but don't go overboard. Look for a style with versatility, particularly if you live in a big city with many different

Ed liked his long hair but wanted to look sexier and better groomed.

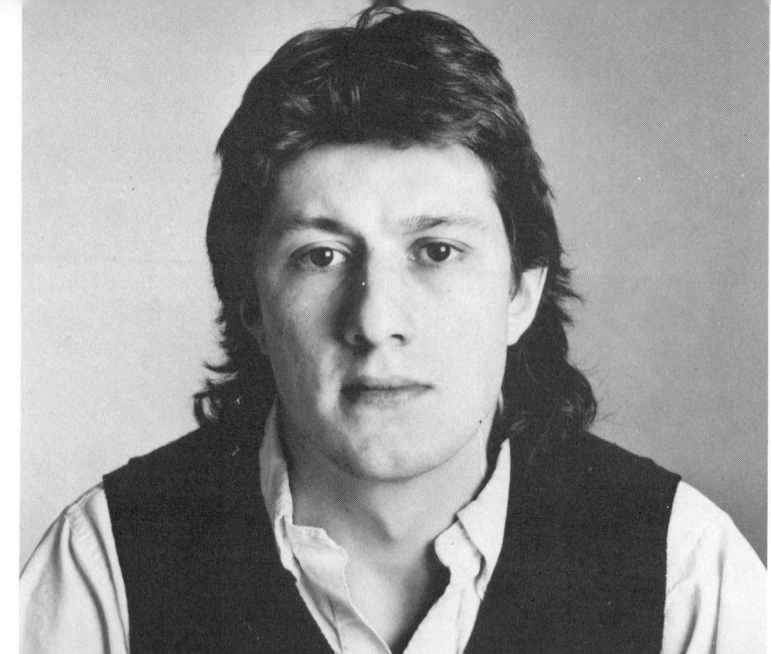

Ed

Ed has medium-textured brown hair. The weight of the longer length made his hair lie flat. I cut his hair short on top and added subtle blond highlights, which visually lengthened his face and elongated his forehead. The short sides work well for most men because they visually widen the eye/cheek area. I kept his hair long in back to strengthen his jawline and give him the feeling he likes of having longer hair. A gel applied to damp hair keeps his hair in shape and gives him the sexy look he wants.

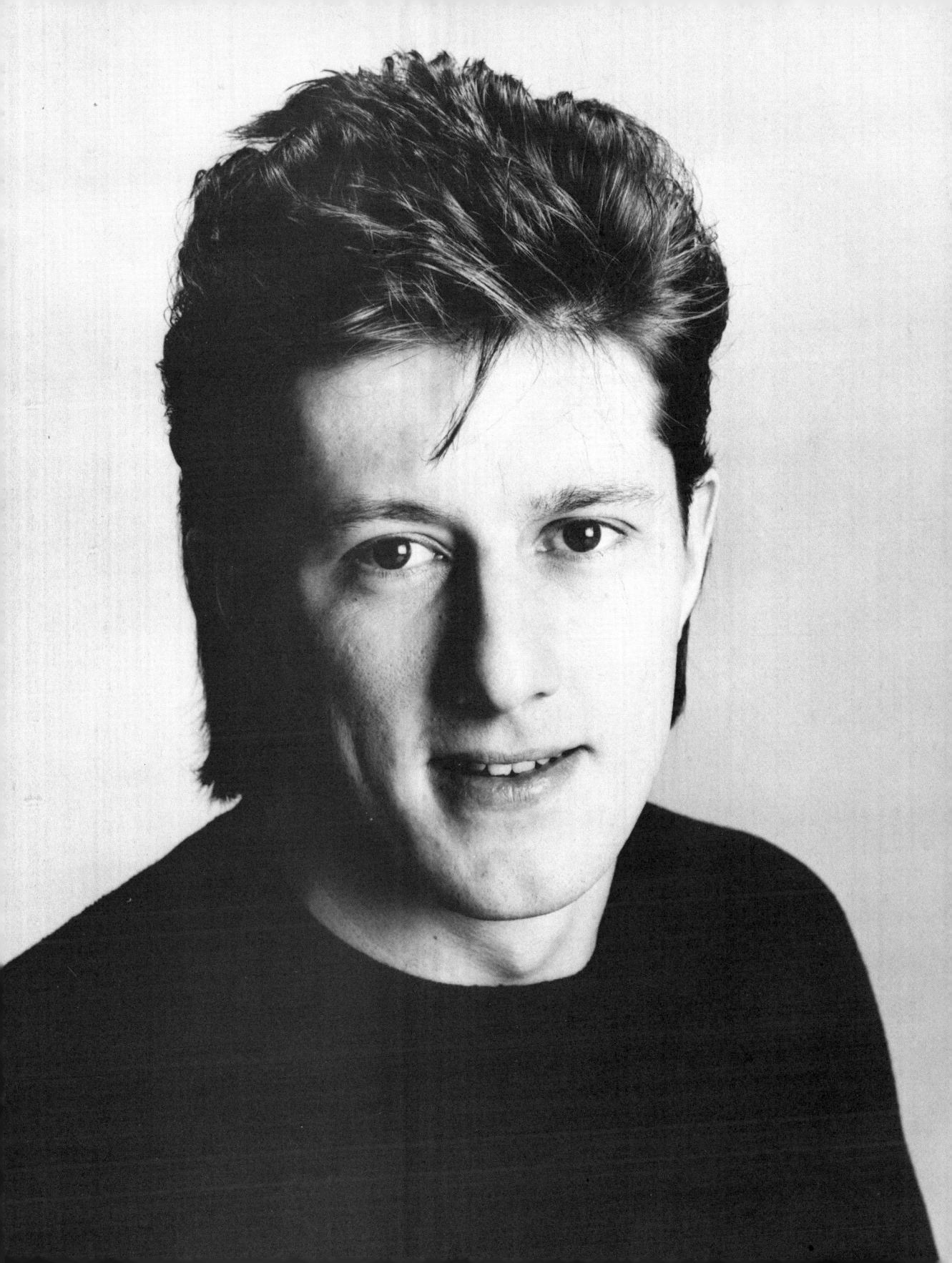

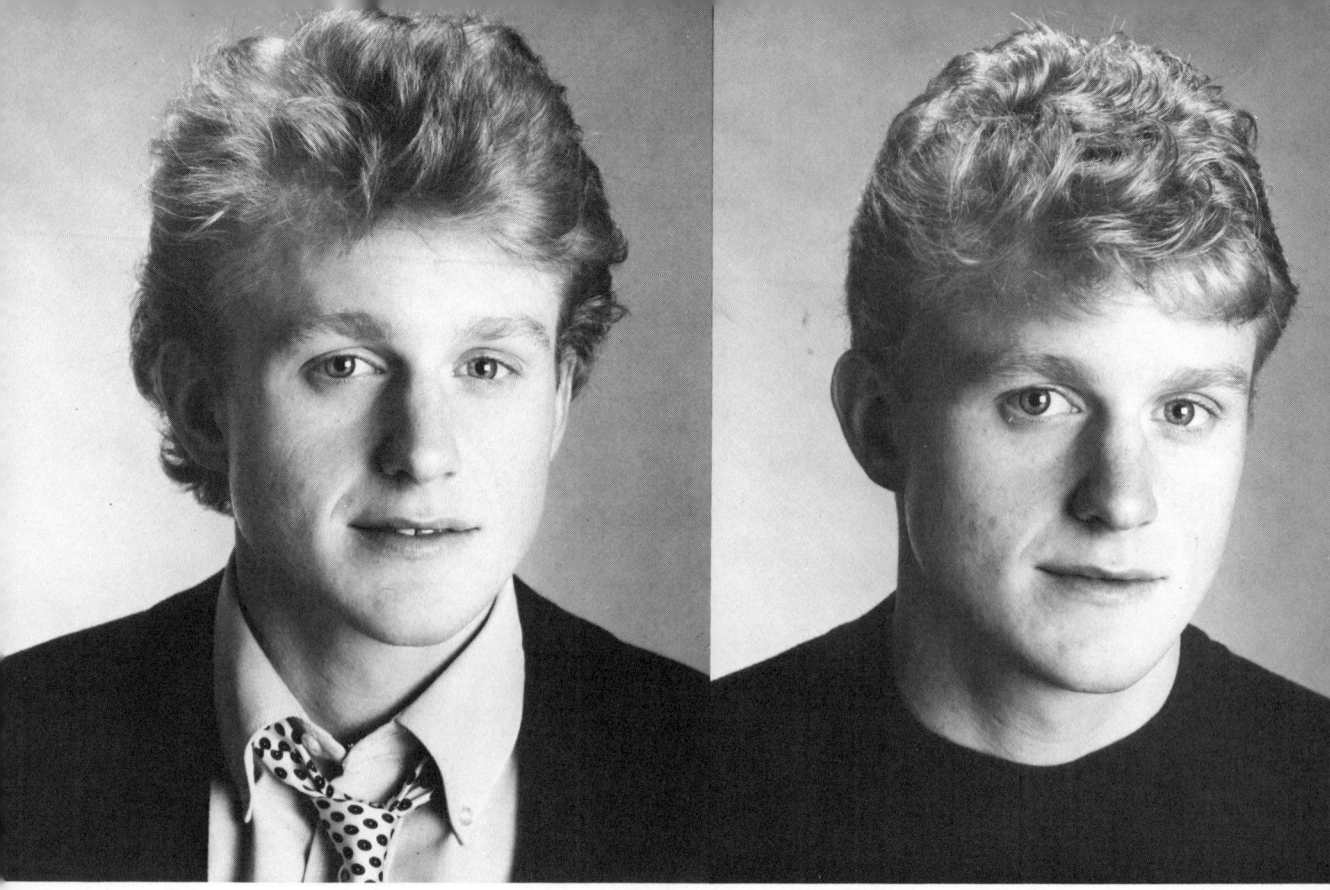

Short, neat hair is classic and shows off a great body and face.

Scott

Scott has fine, blond wavy hair. The weight of his longer hairstyle made it look even thinner. The short tousled cut adds bulk and volume. Lightly groomed with a mousse and dried naturally, his short cut takes only four minutes a day to maintain.

business and social atmospheres. Green punk streaks just won't do for a formal dinner party.

In the creative fields, you usually can grow a moustache or a beard without worrying about office codes, so experiment with many hair lengths and coloring. The point is not to limit yourself. You're in the enviable position of having free rein with your looks. Take advantage of it.

The Goal for the Athlete's Hair

I hope sports are a major part of your life, and not just the Monday night football games on TV. If you jog every day, swim, ski, work out, you must take that activity into consideration when planning your haircut. Active sports make special demands on your hair:

- **Styling.** A short cut is usually best, Bjorn Borg notwithstanding. You'll need a haircut that can go from the shower to the office fast. Short cuts are also easier to keep trimmed and in condition.
- **Condition.** If you expose your hair to harsh elements—sun, wind, cold or hot weather—you'll need to condition it every time you wash it, applying special products to protect it from sun and pool chemicals.

On the other hand, your cut can show off that great body, really play up your physique. And a style with movement in the hair, say a bit longer on top, can look great while you perform.

How Your Hair Can Make You Look Younger

While it's true that in the '80s we may be putting too great an emphasis on youth, it's also true that we have become better at preserving a

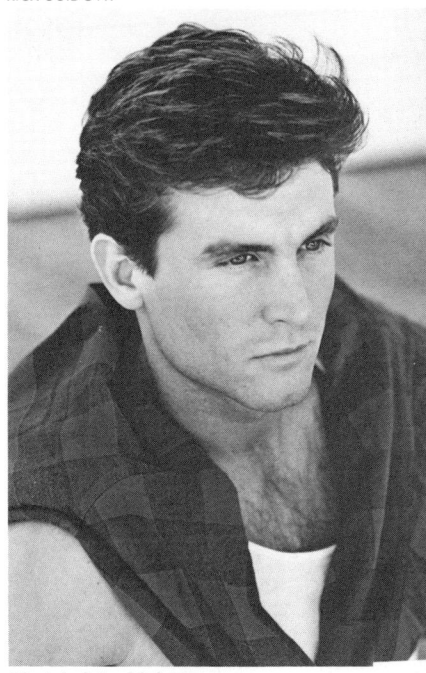

RICK GUIDOTTI

Model: John Maloney

71

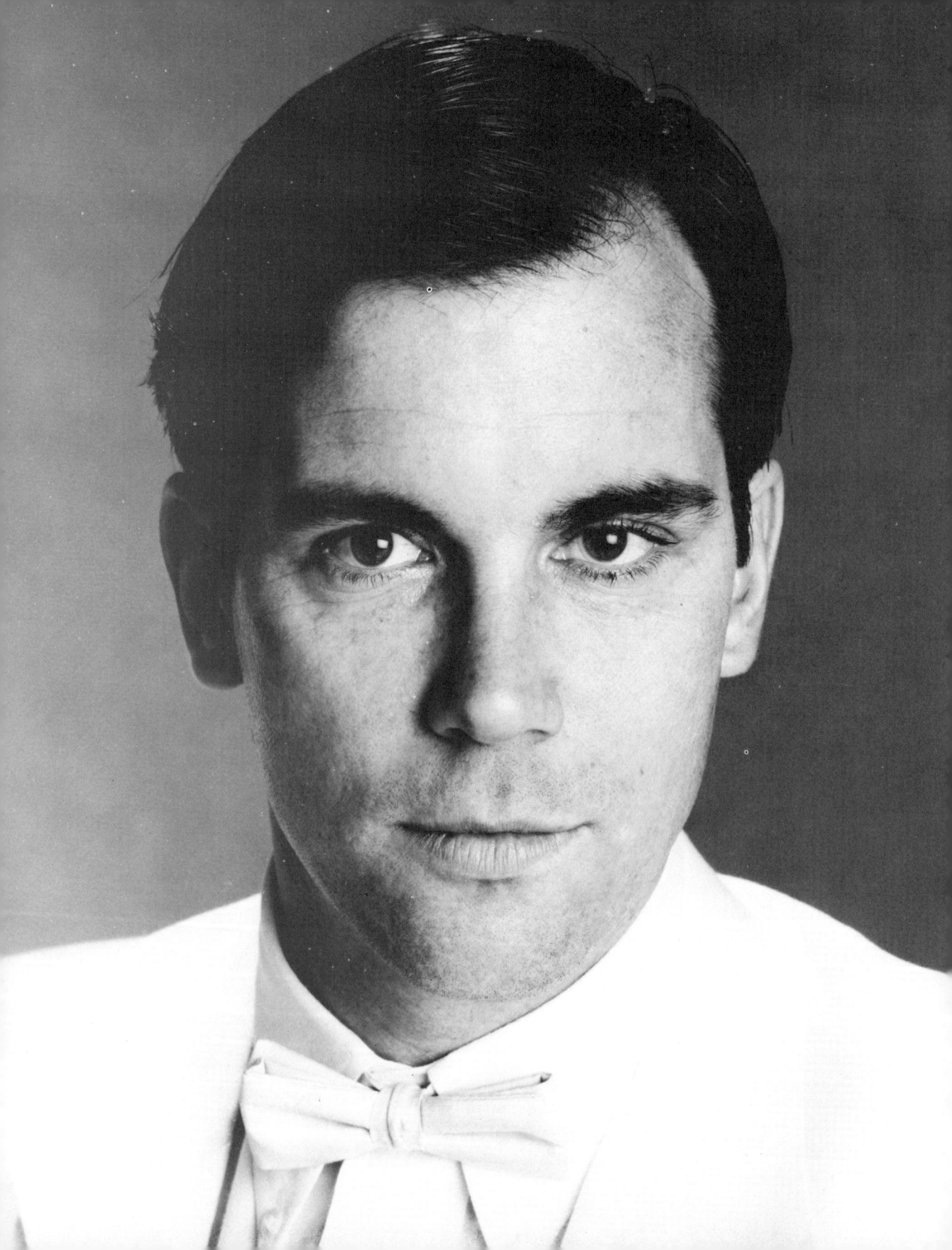

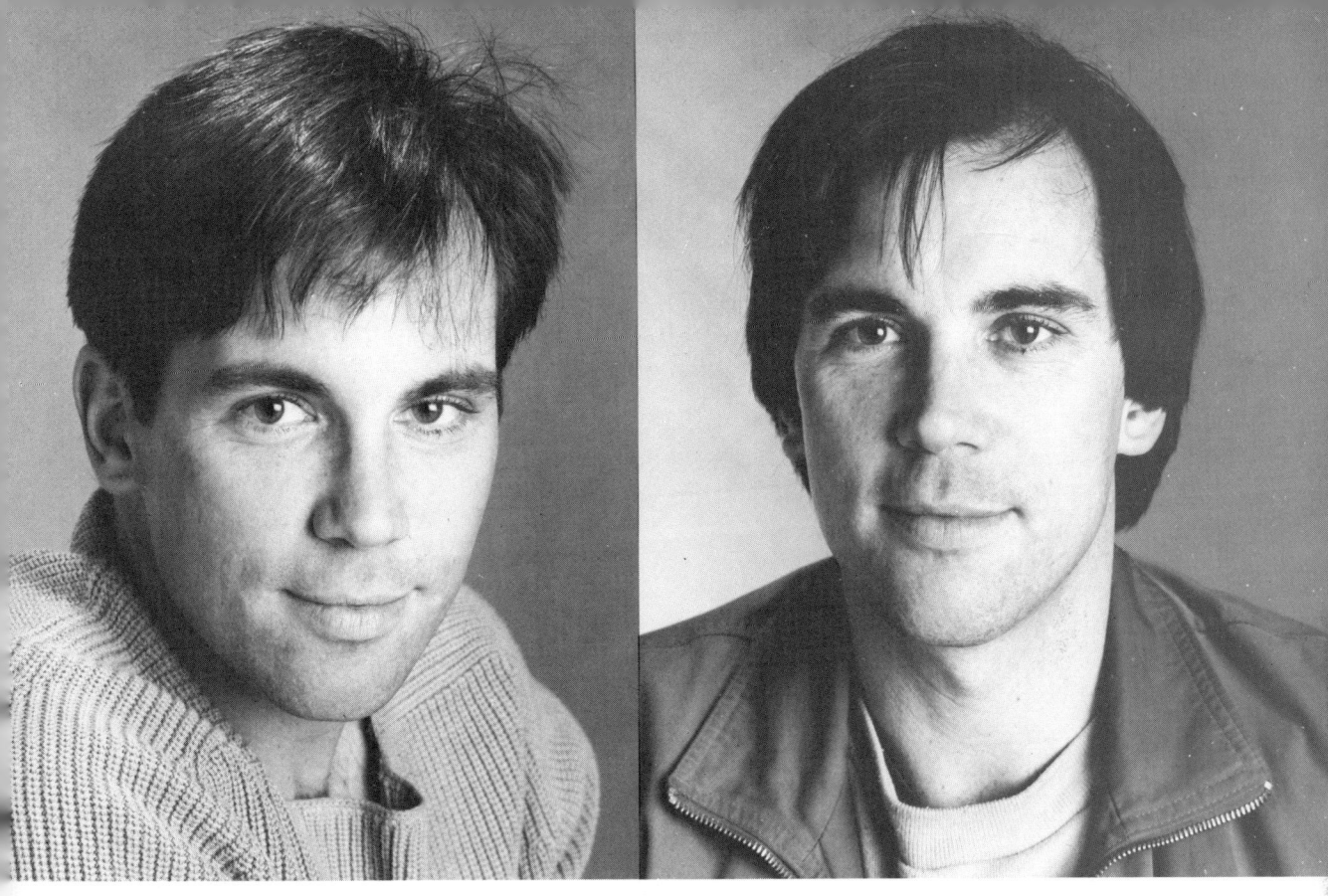

Randy

Why hide your hairline? It could give you dignity and class. I cut Randy's hair shorter all over, which adds bulk to thinning hair. For a casual look, Randy shampoos, uses a finishing rinse, and blow-dries his hair—no combing or brushing needed. For a sophisticated look, he applies gel to damp hair and combs into place.

Randy makes the most of his receding hairline by showing it off.

youthful, healthy appearance than ever before.

One of the most telling signs of age is gray hair. The quickest method of paring years off your appearance is to color your hair a lighter shade of its original color with semipermanent hair coloring. This will cover the gray, add some interesting highlights to your hair, and add shine, too.

As you age, your face develops more character, due to the well-defined lines and bone structure that emerge. Sometimes these lines can be too harsh, making you look older than you really are. The mistake many older men make is to keep wearing their hair in the slicked-back style that looked so good when they had more hair. Dark, flat hair accentuates unflattering facial lines, but such lines can be softened with the right hair. If you have deep lines in your face, you should wear your hair in a looser, fuller style. (Leonard Bernstein is a good example of how a looser, fuller haircut softens facial lines.)

As we age our hair loses some of the color pigment and oil that make it look shiny and healthy. If your hair looks nondescript, you can liven it up easily and undetectably with the semipermanent color wash just mentioned.

How to Look Older and More Authoritative

Yes, there are perfectly good reasons for wanting to appear older.

● You may have a baby face and feel uncomfortable because you don't look as mature as your peers.

● You may be up for a job that usually would go to a senior man—you have the qualifications, but

For social events or job prospects, you may want to look older.

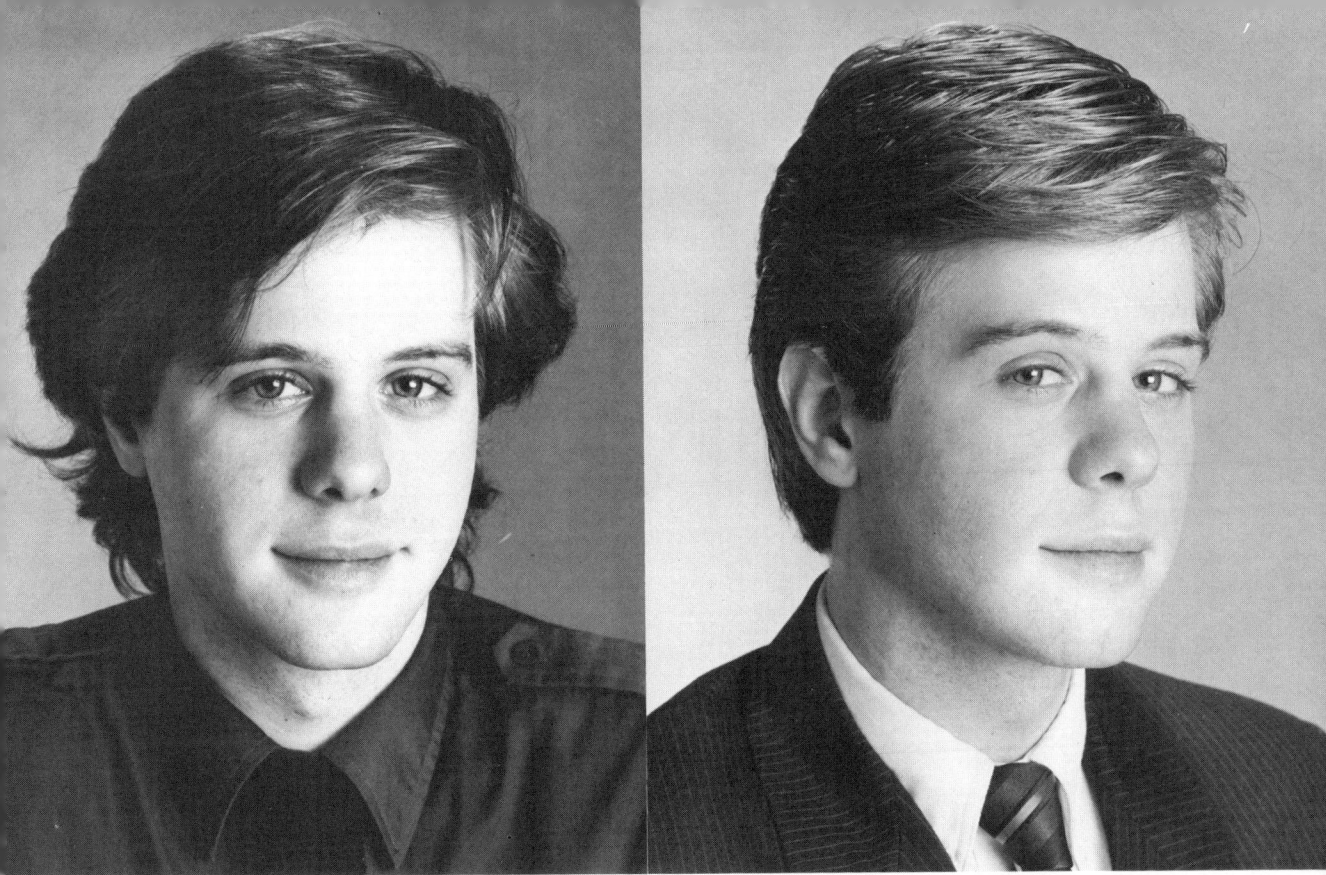

you need to look the part, too.

● You like to think of yourself as an intellectual and feel an older look would fit better with your personality.

You have two options.

The first is to grow facial hair. A moustache, beard, or both will make you seem older, providing an aura of strength and wisdom. As we age, our facial hair becomes thicker, so an association between facial hair and age has developed over the centuries.

The second option is to darken your hair. Darker hair is more authoritative; if you're young and have light-colored hair, you are usually, if unfairly, deemed not as responsible as if your hair were a few shades darker.

Blaine

A well-groomed appearance and a neat, sharp haircut adds age and sophistication here. I cut Blaine's hair to a medium length, giving him the neat on-the-job look but still allowing him a versatile casual style for his private life. A side-part and a groomer keep his hair in place.

75

Celebrities constantly change their hair to project different images.

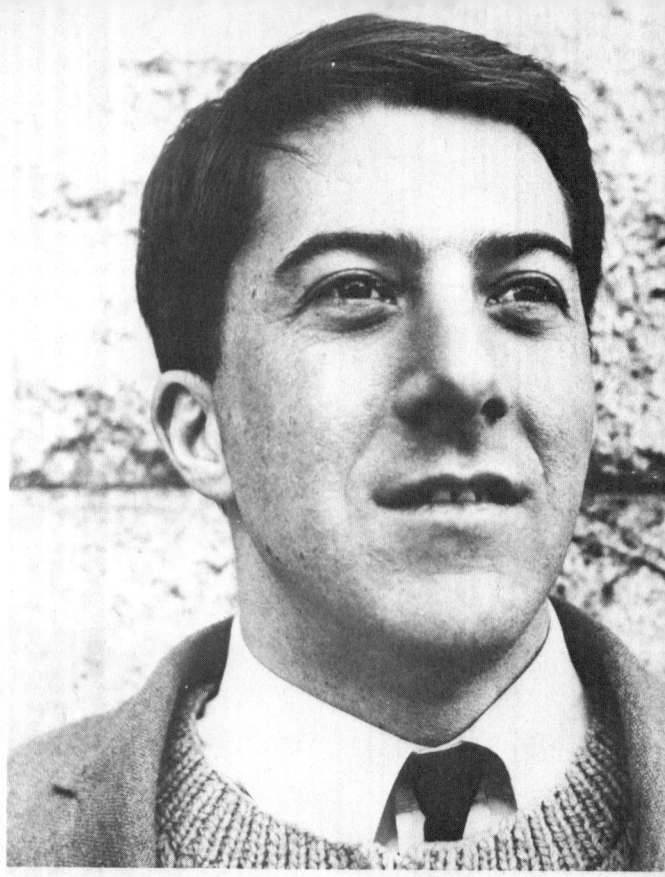

In the '60s, Dustin Hoffman portrayed a student in the award-winning film, The Graduate. His short, preppy brush cut helped project the naive character he played. In real life, Dustin wears his hair medium length. The look is soft, casual, sexy, and much more worldly-wise. Dustin has medium-textured shiny brown hair that adapts to many different looks.

Since we first met John Lennon in the early '60s, his hair set the trend of the times. These three photos reflect the evolution of his look and his many-faceted character. As his personality grew and changed, his hair served to visually reinforce his opinions and his lifestyle. I can't help but wonder what his look would have been today.

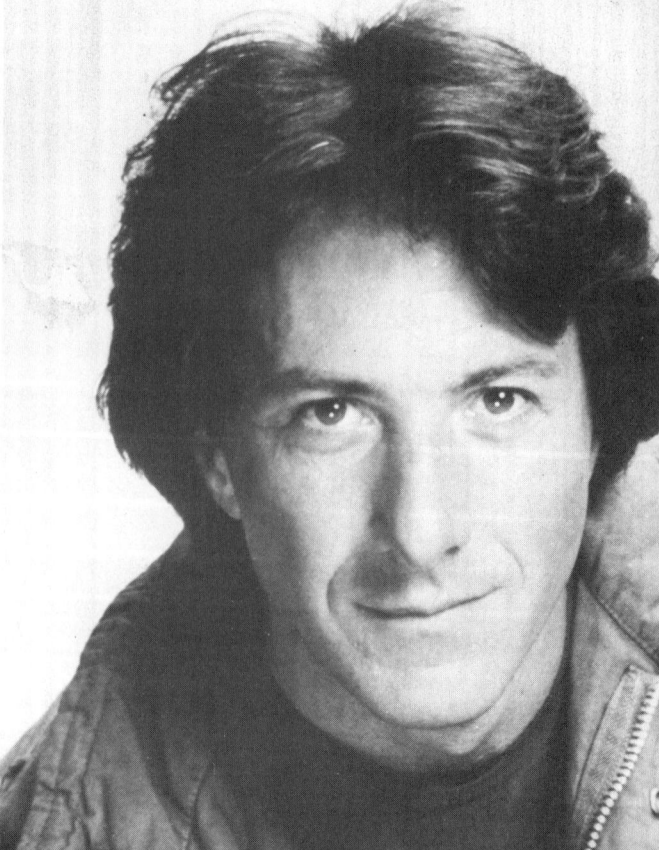

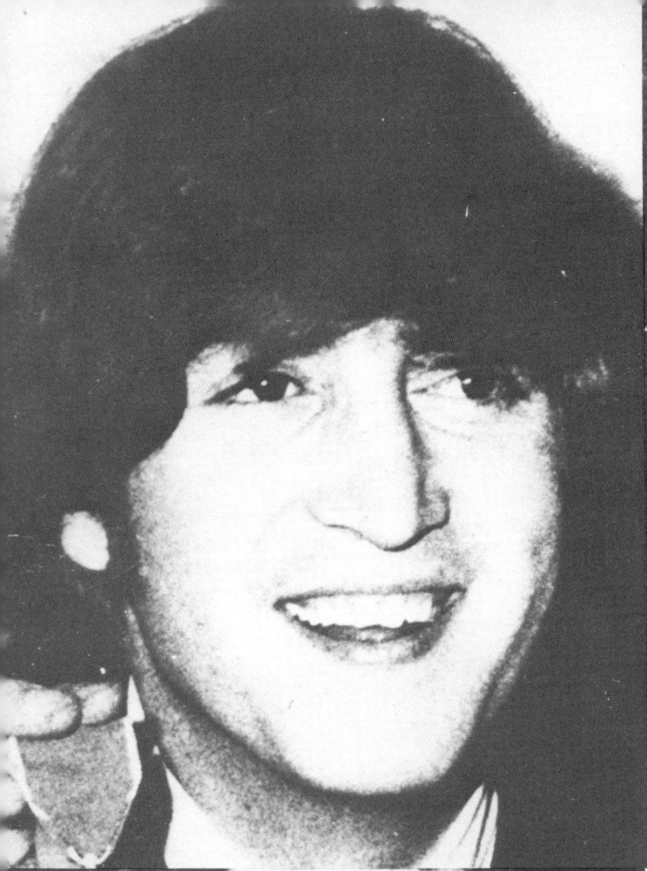

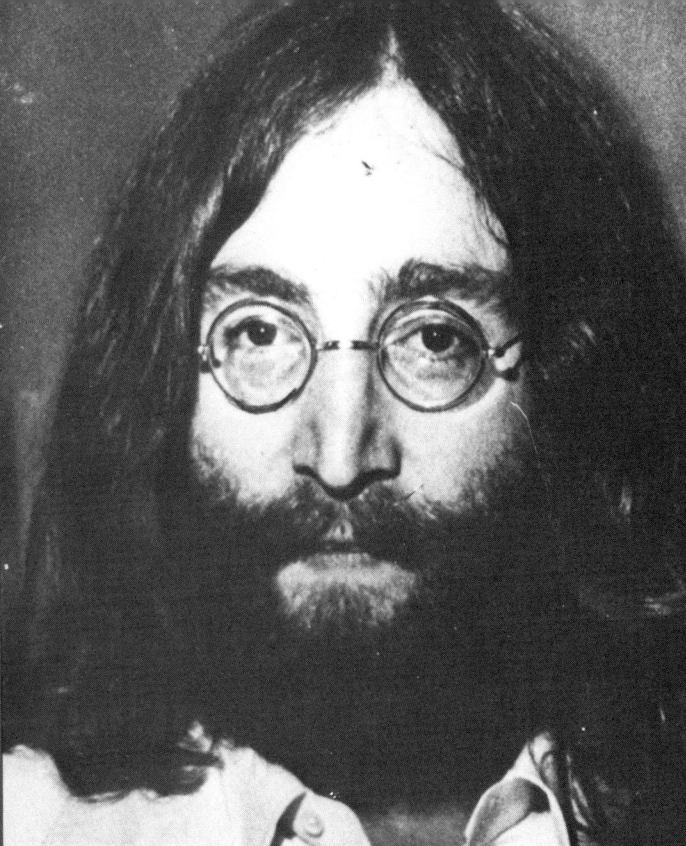

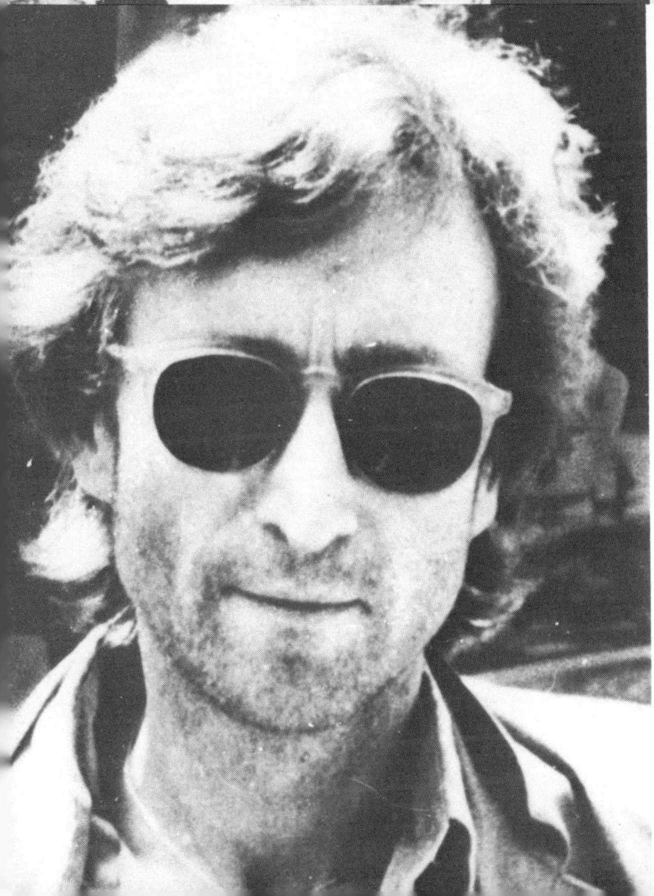

From Beatle haircut to hirsute rebel to final maturity, control, and style.

AP/WIDE WORLD PHOTOS

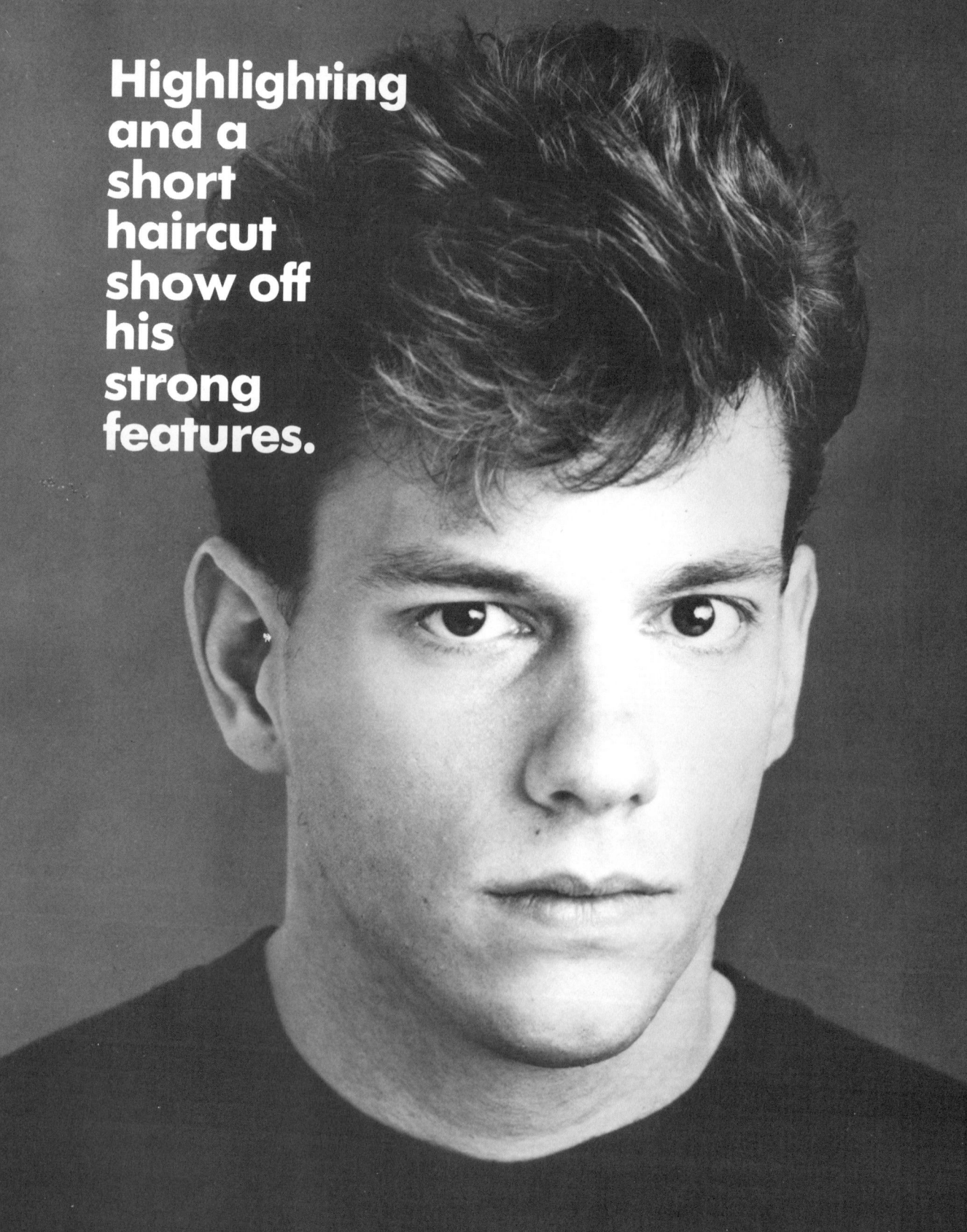

Highlighting and a short haircut show off his strong features.

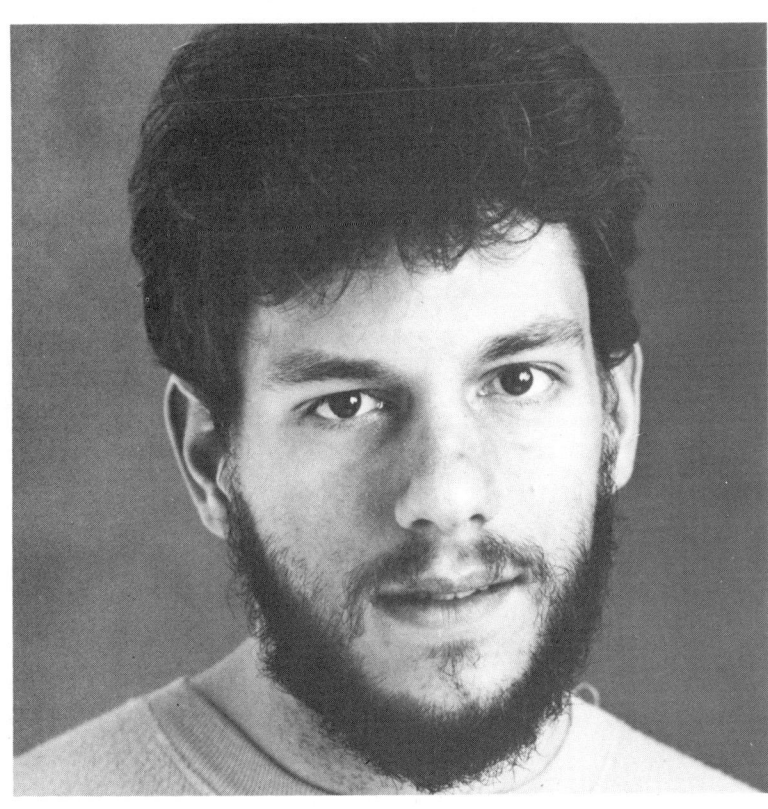

Greg didn't need facial hair.

Greg

"As a New York City casting agent, I need to look neat, professional, and with-it. I was shocked at what a few easy changes could do! George reevaluated my hair qualities and my facial features and changed my outlook too."

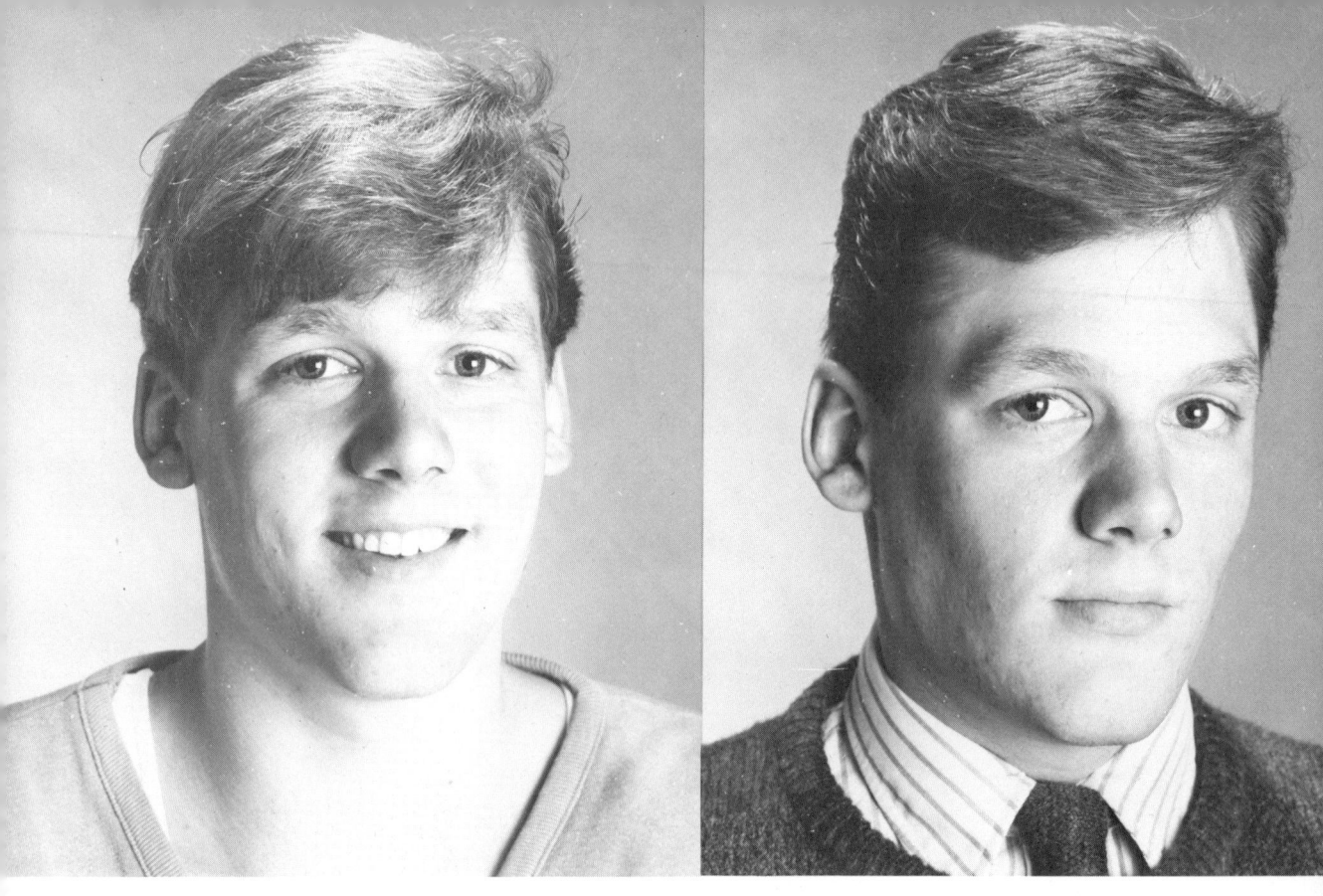

Any haircut can have at least two different looks.

John

John looks rugged, young, and boyish with full, tousled hair. But on the job, he needs a cool, controlled look. The transformation is easy. Freshly shampooed, towel-blotted hair is slicked with styling gel or mousse. He shapes it with a large-toothed comb and it's that simple!

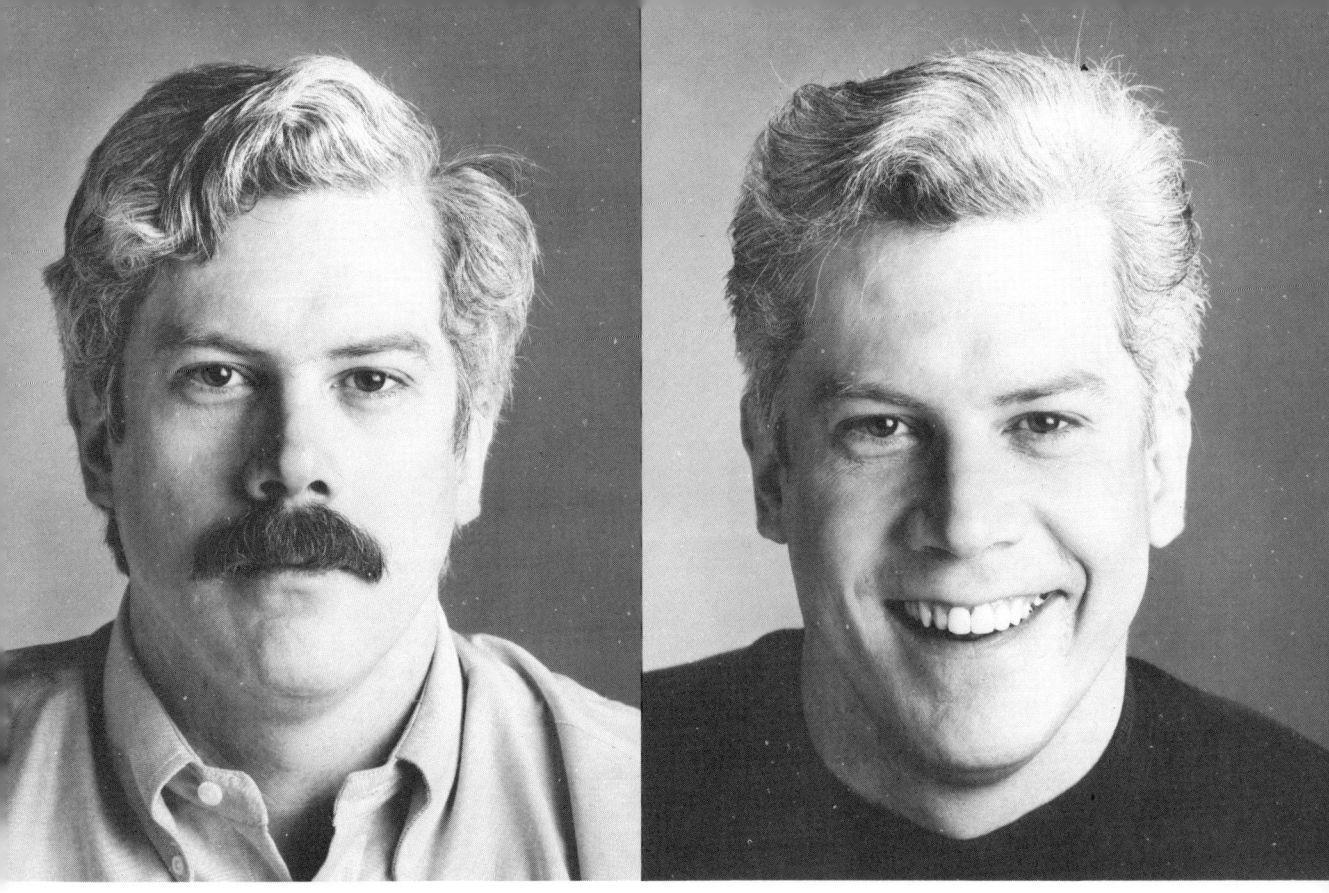

Paul

Paul had worn the moustache for fifteen years. He grew it in college but recently decided to rediscover his face. For a few moments, he felt lost without the moustache but then delighted at the enhanced impact of his smile. A shorter, thinned-out haircut removed bulk and added definition. He looks years younger.

Paul's moustache was a college habit that now added years to his look.

81

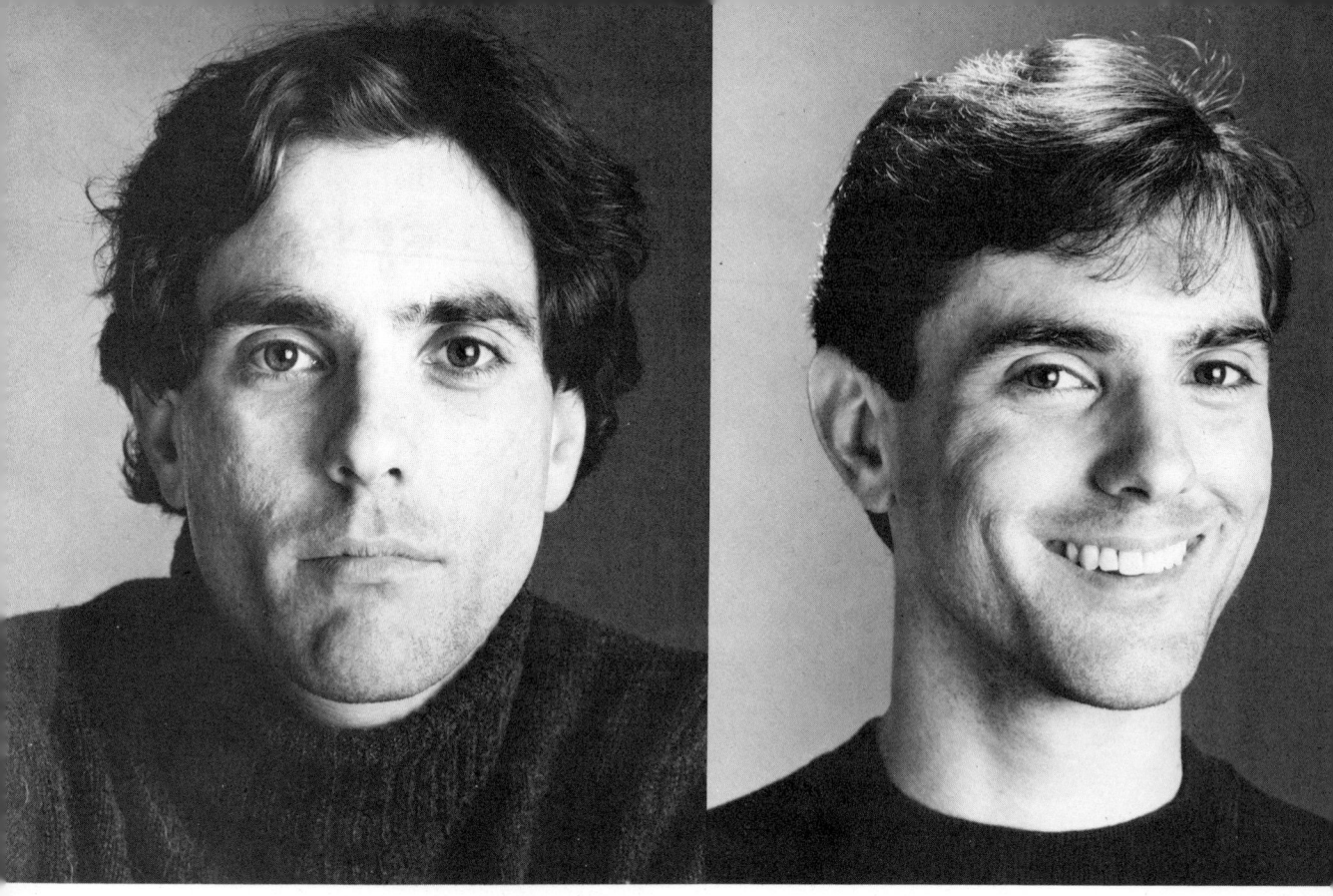

Jack needed height on top, not width at the sides. We changed proportions.

Jack

Jack's long hair in back detracted from his two best facial features: his expressive eyes and warm smile. I cut his hair shorter in back to lift the visual focus away from his neck to his face. Short sides show off his cheekbones and eyes. The forehead tousle softens his hairline.

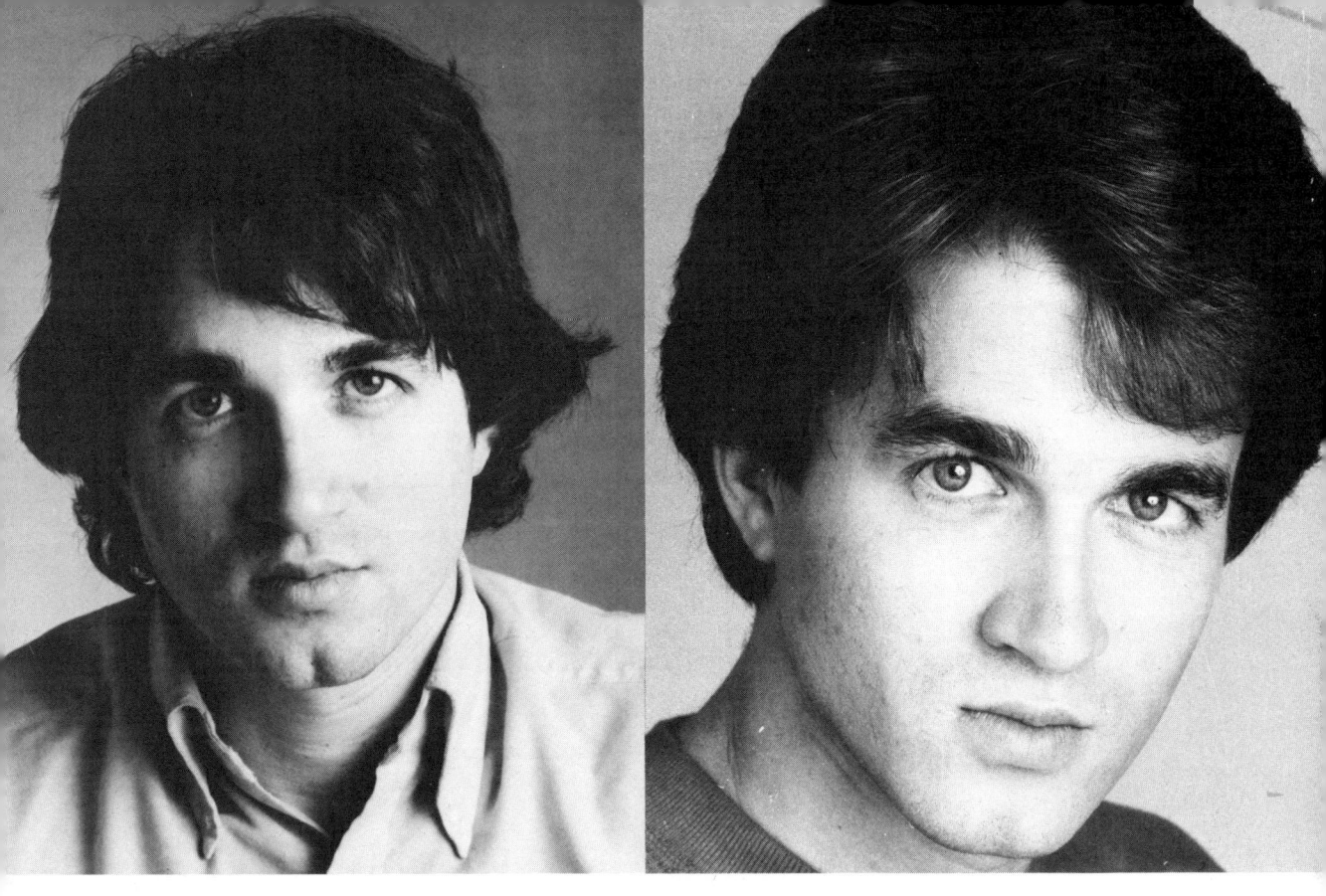

Artie

Long hair detracted from Artie's blue eyes and his dramatic cleft chin. Shorter hair at the nape gives the illusion of a longer neck and exposes his jawline. The close-cropped sides and soft diagonal fall of hair over his forehead play up his eyes. His medium-textured hair requires little styling maintenance. He applies a nonoily hair groomer to damp hair and uses his fingers to style into shape.

The right haircut will bring out your strong points.

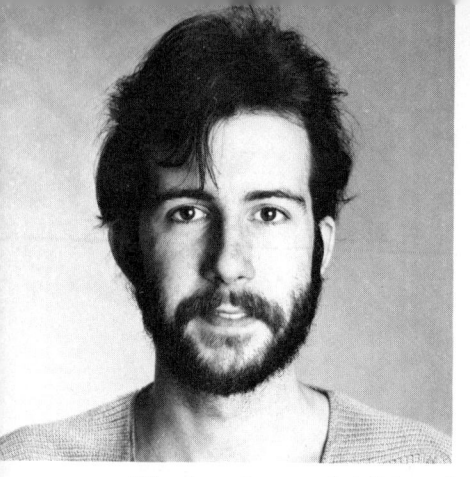

The long hair and full beard were more appropriate for a college town than for B.W.'s new life on Madison Avenue. One option was to pull B.W.'s long hair back to show what he would look like with short hair and a beard. This draws the emphasis up more toward his eyes.

B.W.

B.W. had three major changes in his life happen at the same time. He turned thirty, moved to New York City, and began a totally different career. We updated his image in several steps, recording all phases with photographs. Here is his own account of the evolutionary process. Each change brought out dramatically different characteristics.

Interview with B.W.

When I turned thirty, it was time for some changes in the way I looked and the way I was living. I had a very successful career as a merchandiser in a college town in North Carolina. I worked freelance for the best stores in town. I was well paid and had a house with a backyard and a garden. Those were the things I gambled with to move to New York.

I had thought about moving to New York for years. Merchandising fulfilled my visual sense, but I wanted to focus on a wider range of design work, and New York is the best place to be if that's your goal.

I was always conscious of my image. If you're going to sell your sense of design to someone,

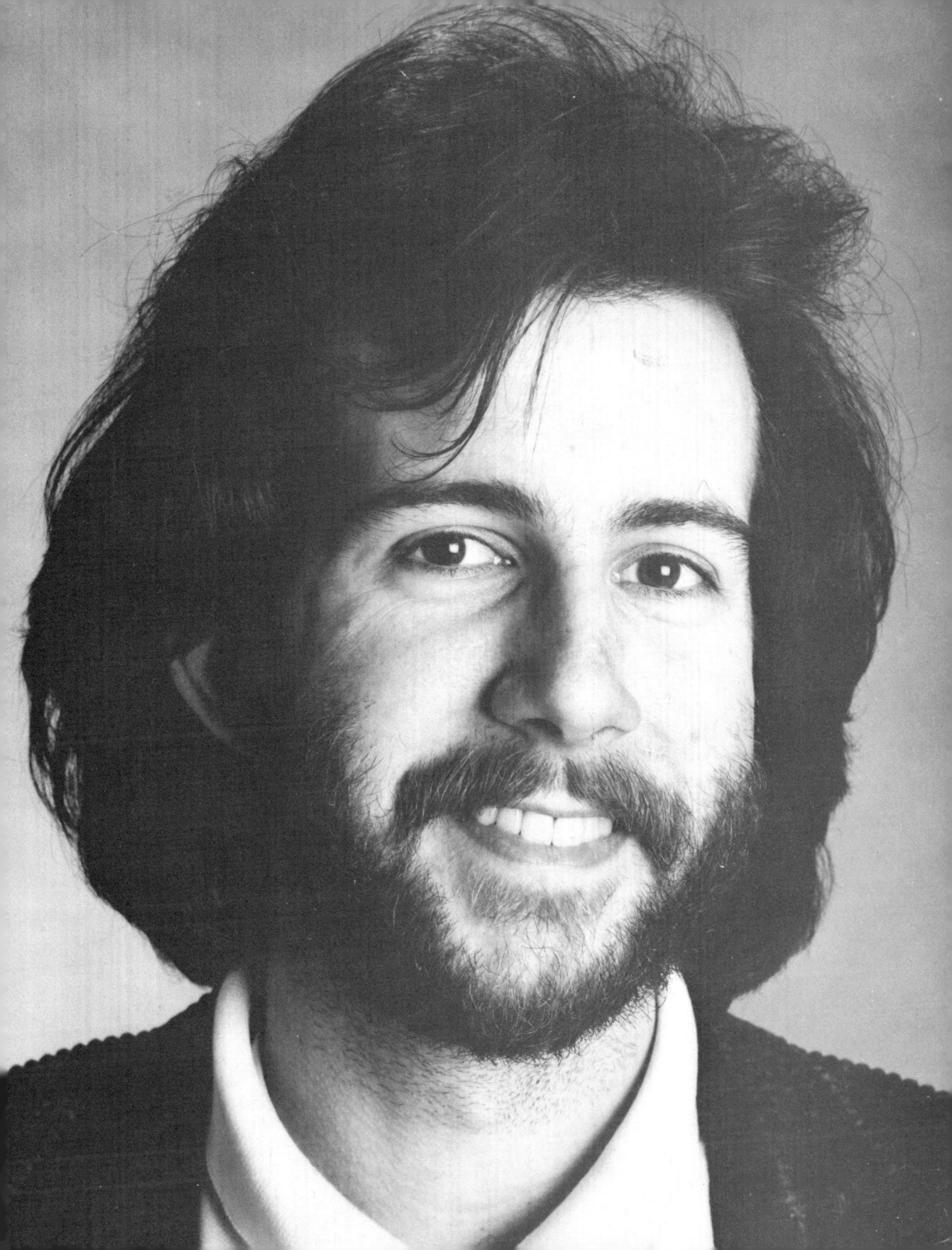

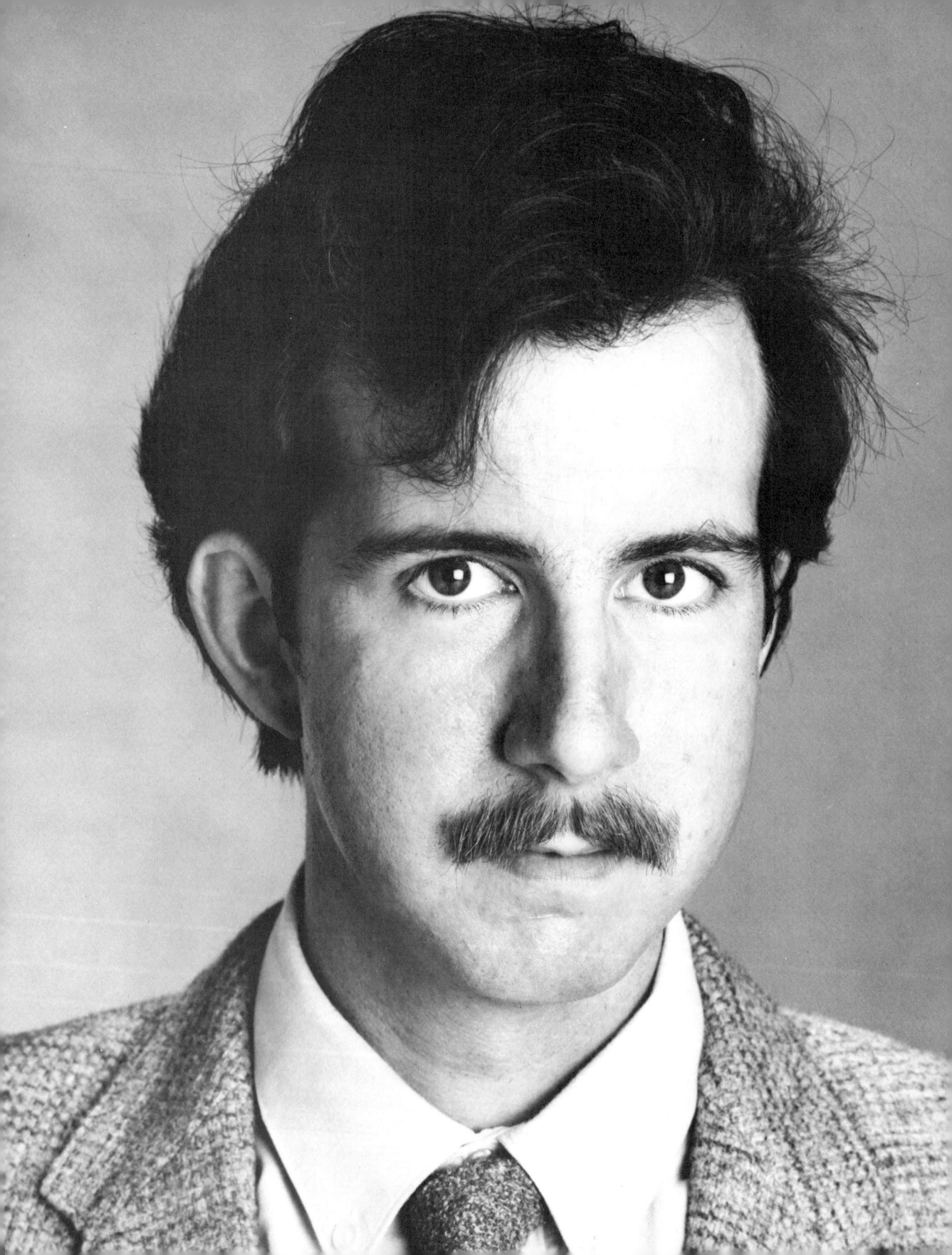

you've got to look right. So I've always cared about the way I looked.

Usually I like to wear my hair medium to long. I figure it probably won't be long before I lose my hair, like my grandfather. So I might as well enjoy it while I've got it. I'm a tactile, sensual kind of person, and I like to run my hands through my hair. It feels thick and sexy and I like the way it moves around. It grabs my hand back and feels good.

I like short hair for another reason—because it is very easy. I don't have to deal with it. I can just wash it and that's it. I condition it just to keep it nice and shiny and soft. I can just get out of a shower and towel my head and go. But short hair makes me feel twelve years old. So I guess I relate it back to when I was a kid.

Longer hair softens the line of my cheekbones and makes my face look better, younger. This haircut is terrific. It waves in the right places. I would like not to use a blow dryer too much on it. Right now it tends to wing out if I don't blow-dry it. George showed me how to dry my hair naturally instead, pushing it upward so it doesn't wing out.

When I came here, my mind was racing a lot. I knew I wanted to make a change in my appearance. For one thing, I wanted to look younger coming to New York at thirty. And I wanted to look a little more professional. If you're dealing with the media, which is what I wanted to do, then you have to be able to sell yourself more, which is a more sophisticated process here than in North Carolina. It helps a great deal to look fresh and with-it.

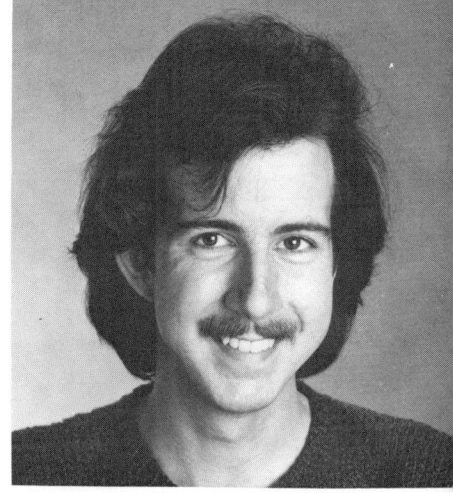

Removing the beard entirely gives his eyes the most impact. Medium-to-short hair length gives him a professional, well-groomed, easily maintained appearance while still leaving enough length to strengthen his jawline.

87

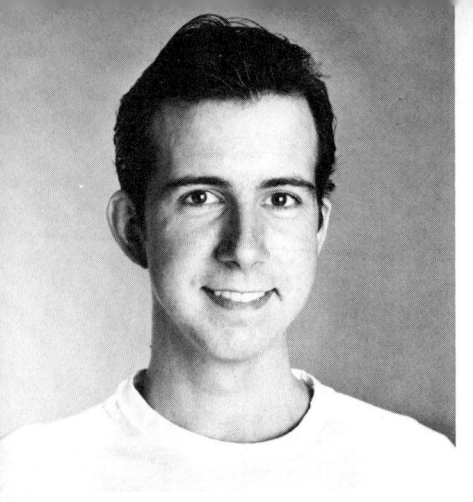

I wanted to present a fresh look to myself as well, so that when I got up in the morning and looked in the mirror, I would realize that, hey, things are different.

I liked the moustache and beard, but I really felt like making a clean sweep. It had been five years since I had seen my real face. Now I can grow a moustache with a whole different attitude—as another option for my looks. I'm not hiding behind it anymore.

After being here only two months, I got a permanent job on *Gentleman's Quarterly,* the leading men's magazine. That boosted my self-confidence. I'm one of only two designers, which is wonderful.

I've started dressing differently, putting clothes together in a more relaxed way. In the South, I tended to dress more preppy, more coordinated. Now I might throw on something I never would have thought of putting together before, just to see what it does, instead of having my eight color-coordinated outfits all in a row.

In North Carolina, I knew what I wanted to look like. There was one look for me. Here, I'm constantly experimenting, depending on the circumstances, the part of the city I'm going to, how I feel that day, who I have to meet. I can go to a different place every day with a different look and feel confident.

Here, first impressions are so important. For anyone to come up to you in the first place, you must be acceptable in some way. Each way you present yourself creates different observations in people, makes them react to you differently. You

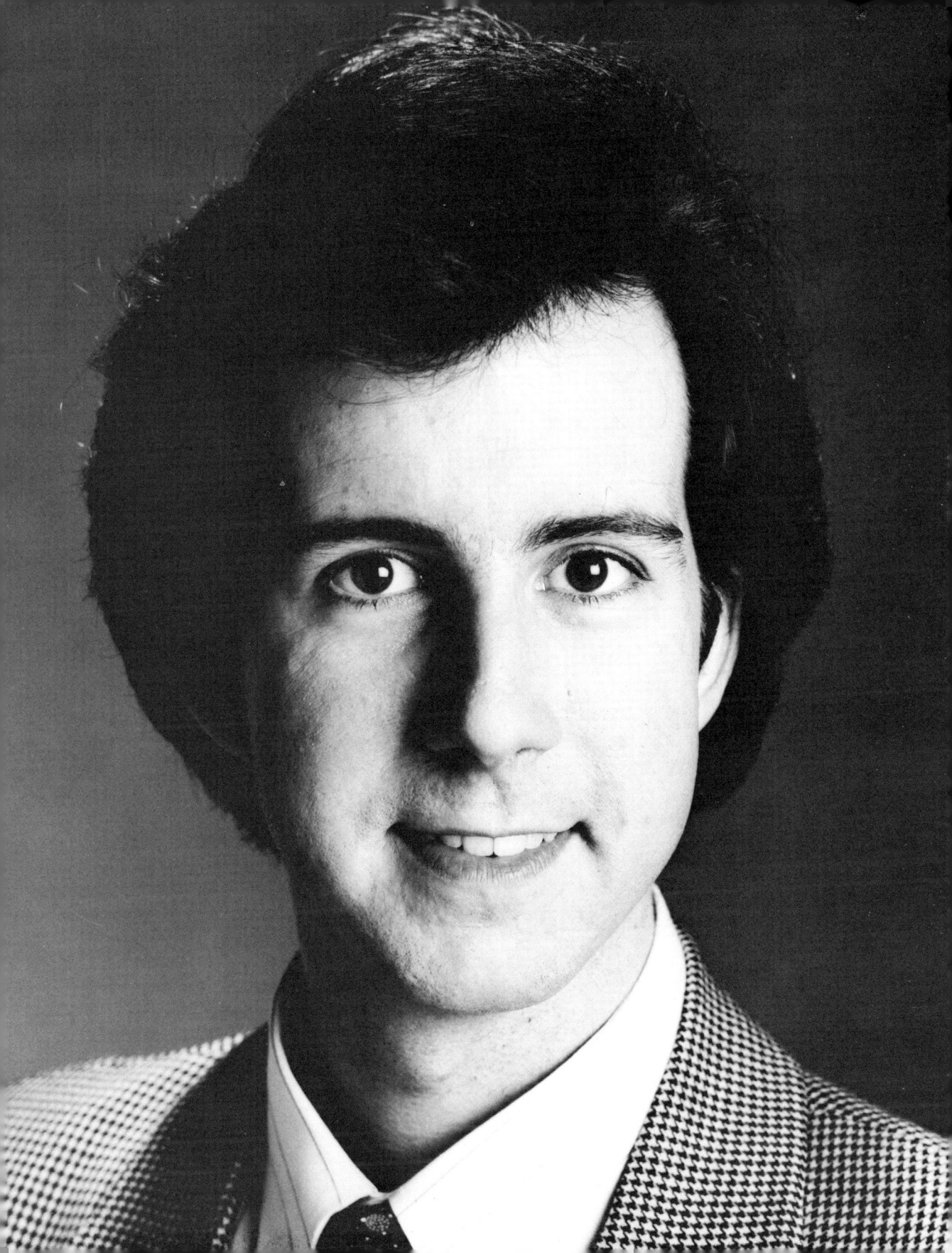

can have five different looks and get five different reactions.

I act differently when I have a beard. The beard gives me a look of authority. The beard also attracts a different type of person. When I'm bearded, people respect me more; they call me "Sir" or "Mister." I'm definitely not a boy. When I'm bearded I'm more huggable. But I get tired of being a teddy bear; I enjoy shaving my face, showing my face.

When I'm clean-shaven, I'm more devil-may-care. People call me "Son." I don't think so much of heavy concerns.

I think you tend to look like the part of yourself that you're most comfortable with at the time. You can look any number of ways if you're comfortable with your looks. And it doesn't look like you're putting on something or someone. It looks like it's just you.

Putting It All Together

Just as no one's life is completely one-dimensional, there is no one rigid look for you. You want hair that will complement all the different characters you play in the course of the day. If you have to look strict sometimes and unrestrained at others you can have hair that will give you the versatility to achieve both looks.

Your hair, your features, your lifestyle—these are the components. Accept the challenge of putting them all together.

5.

HOW TO GET A GREAT HAIRCUT

Use What You Know to Create a Partnership with Your Hair Stylist

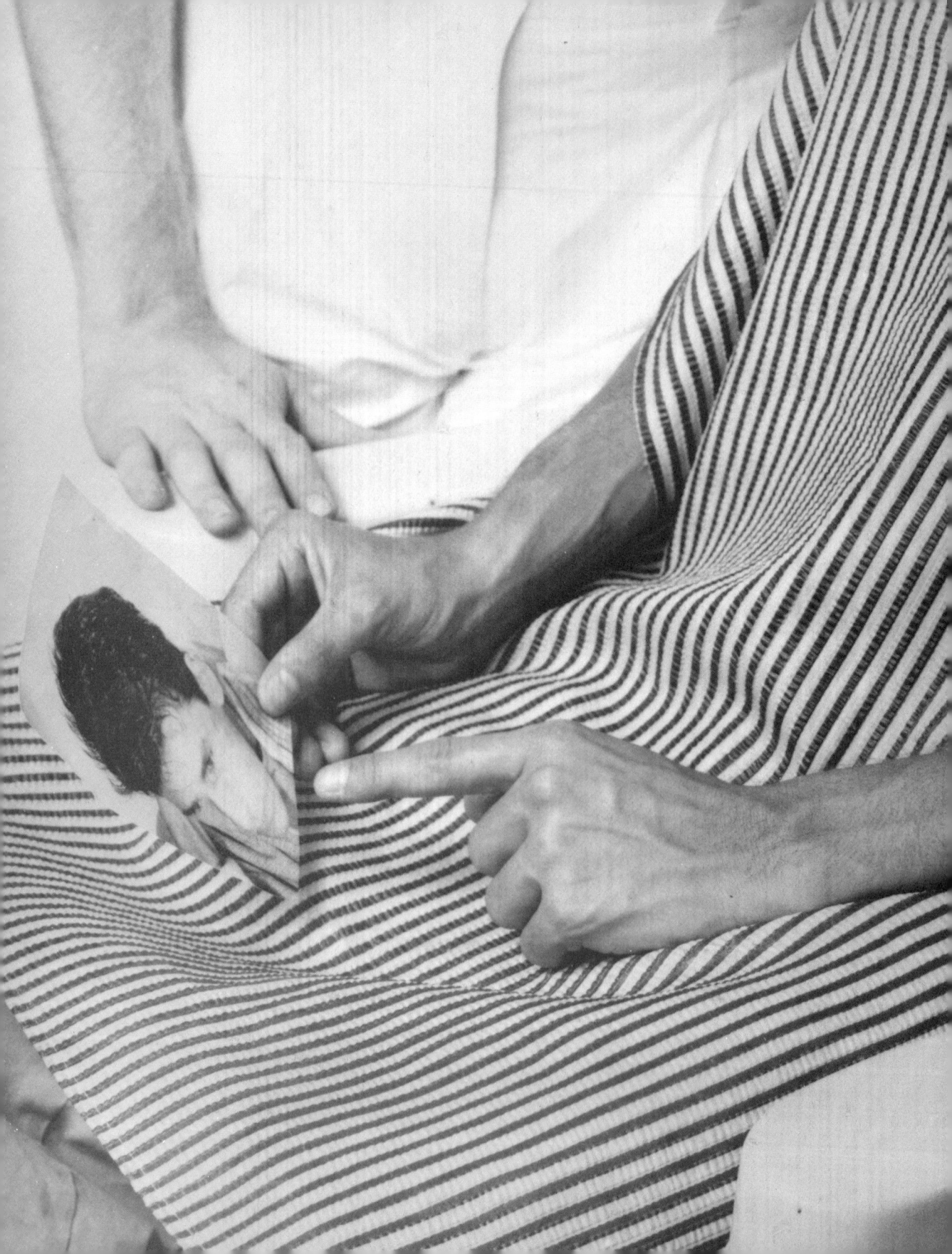

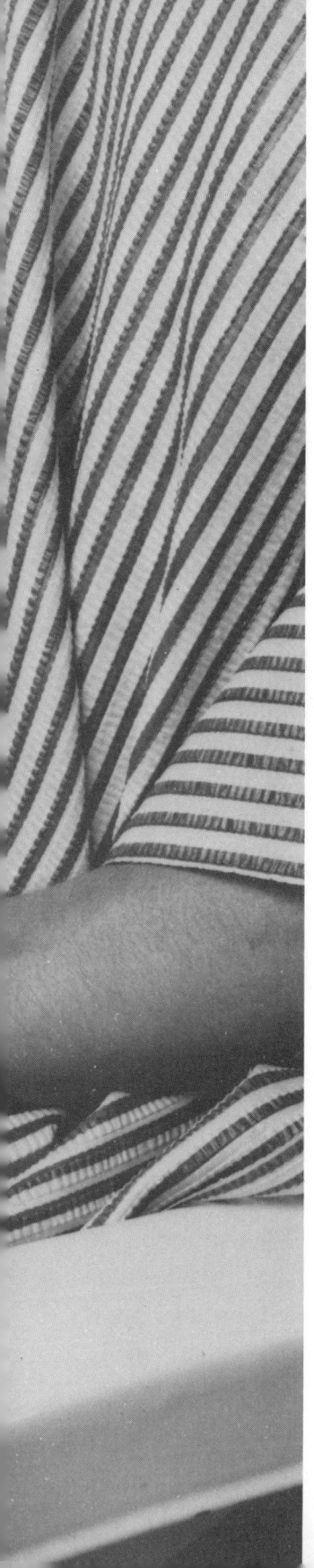

It's Up to You

You've spent most of this book learning about your looks and what a great haircut can do for you. Now it's time to get one. But before you select a stylist and take action, let's review what you know so far. You're going to take this knowledge with you to the barbershop or salon.

Remember, *you're* in charge. "But I'm going to an expert. Shouldn't the stylist control the situation?" you may well ask. Your hair cutter is there to work *with* you on a haircut that shows you at your very best. Rather than placing yourself totally in another's hands, you can create a true partnership with the knowledge you have now. You will be giving your cutter real, helpful guidance (and he'll respect you for it) that will make his job easier and leave *both* of you well satisfied. Best of all, you'll like your looks and yourself better.

Now we'll go back over the points we covered in the first chapters, but this time you're going to make some decisions with an eye to that all-important first meeting with the person who will execute your wishes.

The Right Haircut for Your Facial Shape

As I mentioned in Chapter 2, there really is no perfect face, and very few men come close to ideal proportions. But for the most flattering look, your

(89%)—

—(11%)

TOO LONG
OTHER

hairstyle should work to bring your face closer to the ideal oval shape. This holds true no matter what the current trend is in men's hair. Your style can be short, medium, or long—the same general shape can be created in any length.

For an oval face: You can wear any hairstyle that brings out your best facial features.

For a round face: Try framing your face with hair combed over about half your forehead, with medium length hair on the sides of the head (two to three inches long). A high part (an inch or inch and a half away from the center of the head) running straight back will help narrow your face. Avoid styles that hug the head or are combed straight back.

For an oblong face: This face shape can be visually shortened with the proper part. Part your hair in line with the outside of your eyebrow, angling it back toward the center of your crown. This also adds an illusion of width to the face and head. Hair falling over half the forehead further shortens an oblong face.

In general, you should avoid hair combed straight back, since such a dramatic style opens up the face, making it appear even longer. Also avoid wearing a bulk of hair on top of the head. Again, this will have a lengthening effect.

For a triangular face: Your face is wider at the jaw than at the forehead, so you will want to add width at the forehead and sides of the head to balance the face's upper and lower sections. A part lined up with the middle of the eyebrow will visually widen this section of your face.

For a heart-shaped face: Your face is wider at the forehead than at the jaw, so you will want to fill in the area where your face narrows, keeping the hair shorter on top. (For example, if hair on the side of your head is two and a half inches long, top hair should be cut about half an inch shorter.) Your part should be one and a half inches from the center of the head, running straight back. Let your hair fall so that it covers about half (or a bit more) of your forehead.

Using Your Hair to Play Up Your Facial Features

Once you have decided on the overall outline of your hair according to your face shape, you can then play up the features you like the most.

Your forehead. Now you must decide how much of your forehead to reveal or cover. This will depend both on your face shape and you other features.

If your hairline is low or you have a good, well-defined hairline, try combing your hair back off the face. This visually lengthens short faces. A part lined up with the middle of your eyebrow, running straight back, also lengthens your face.

If you have a receding hairline, you can cover your losses by combing some hair across the fore-head. But please don't try parting hair near the ear and swirling it around the crown to simulate a full crop. You fool no one.

If your forehead is narrow, part your hair farther down your head and angle the part toward the center of your crown to widen the face visually. (Line up your part with the outside of your eye-brow.)

Wide foreheads need narrowing. You can do this by parting the hair closer to the center of your head or by letting a tousle fall over your forehead, breaking the expanse of skin.

Your eyebrows. You can darken wispy or lightly colored eyebrows to add definition to your eyes and interest to your face. Most men have medium-thick, medium-dark eyebrows, which is fine. Very heavy brows look best when hair is worn off the face.

Your eyes. Hair falling on the forehead directs attention to the eyes (but never wear full "Dutch boy" bangs). To play up your eyes even more, keep hair short on the sides of the head and keep your sideburns short, too. This opens up the face, and the eyes become more important.

Ideally, the space between your eyes should be the length of one eye. If you feel your eyes are too close together, move your part farther to the side of your head to widen the face.

Your cheekbones. High cheekbones are most desirable. They give added impact and more drama to the face. They stand out from the face, above the cheeks, giving the face a sculpted look. (They are much more noticeable on people with slimmer faces.)

If your cheeks are rounded, you can still get some of the benefit of high cheekbones by using your sideburns. Sideburns are important because they act like small arrows to point at your cheekbones. The more prominent the cheekbones, the more powerful the face looks.

To maximize your cheekbones, your sideburns should be cut even with the top of the bone. Your cheekbones will look wider.

To cut down your cheekbones and slim your face, wear your sideburns just hitting the bottom of the bone.

Your nose. To minimize a large nose, wear a hairstyle that attracts attention elsewhere. Wear bulk on *top* of the head, since large noses tend to make the top of the head look too flat. Shorter hair at the sides will distract attention from your nose to your cheekbones. Balance the prominent nose in profile with longer hair in the back of the head.

If your nose is small, shorter hair overall will make it and your other facial features more pronounced.

Your ears. First decide if your ears look too large or small, after comparing them with the proportions of your face and head as a whole. If they are too large or stick out, wear fuller hair on the sides of your head, behind your ears, filling in the distance between the tops of your protruding ears and your head.

Your lips. Playing up your mouth or minimizing its flaws is best done with facial hair.

Your chin and jaw. You can fill in a narrow, pointed chin by growing hair longer and thicker behind the ears, so it shows below the earlobe and fills in the lower third of your face.

Facial hair is your best cosmetic for building up, cutting down, hiding, reshaping, or dramatizing this section of your face.

Ponder what a beard could do for you.

Your neck. If your neck is short and wide, short hair is best. It should be cut in a V shape in back. Wear a style with more hair on top of the head. Top height makes the neck appear slimmer than it actually is.

If your neck is long and thin, slightly longer hair—a half inch or more below your shirt collar—is best. Instead of a V, hair in back should be cut straight across or in a U shape.

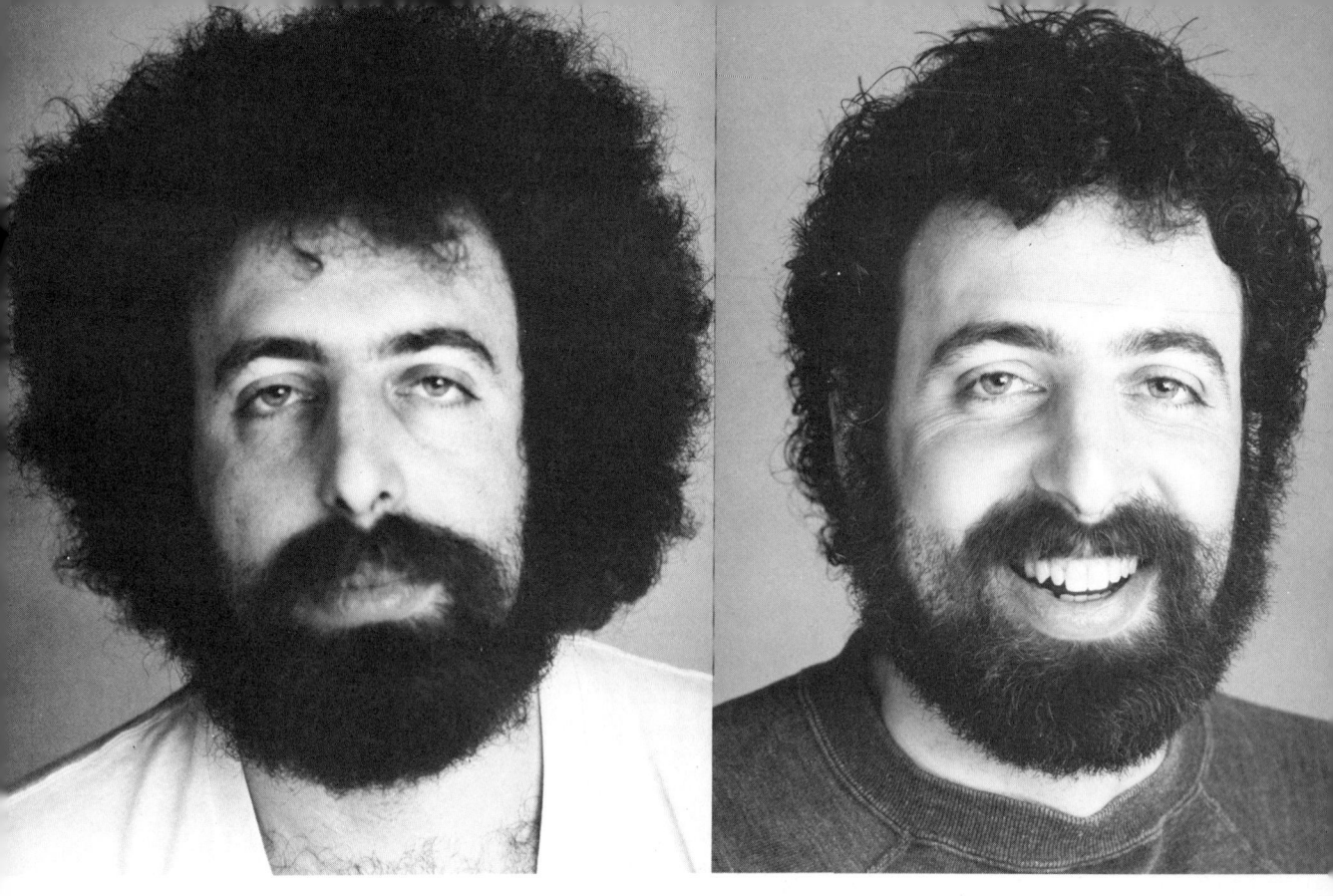

Allen

Allen's personality finally emerges from under a bushel of hair.

Thick, frizzy, dry curly hair and a dry, overgrown, out-of-shape beard were Allen's problems. Conditioning his hair constantly made it soft, shiny, and wavy. The shape of his new cut now complements his face, widening it by showing some ear and esthetically balancing his beard. His new look is sexy, easy, and yet more in control.

Working with Your Type of Hair

In Chapter 3, we looked at four characteristics of your hair: its texture, condition, amount, and formation. Your hair must make the most of these characteristics in order to look its best.

Your Hair's Texture

Fine Hair. A good precision cut is especially important for you. Fine hair shows every cutting mistake, every wrong angle of the scissors. So choose the person who cuts your hair with great care.

Your best general haircut is one that is short on the sides and back but longer on top. Your stylist can cut the longer hair on top to fall in a pleasing way.

Using a hair groomer to comb fine hair straight back is a good option if you have strong facial features to show off. (Hair combed straight back accentuates facial features.) The exception here is if you have a narrow face. A combed-back style will accentuate that even more. Thin faces need thicker hair on the sides of the head to balance them. If your facial features are angular (like Leonard Nimoy's), combing your fine hair back will only increase the angles you want to soften.

The length you wear fine hair depends on the amount of hair you have. The more hair you have, the longer you can wear it. But remember to keep it clean and in good condition. Fine hair shows excess oil and dirt fast! If you want the look of thick, full hair, you will need a routine like the one I devised for David Frost (see Chapter 1). This is taking for granted that you have a good basic cut.

Medium texture. This is the most versatile hair.

You can wear it in straight or wavy styles, short or long.

Coarse texture. Steely-textured hair will hold a shape and stay put in a breeze. It's very easy to care for. But it looks best in short-to-medium length. It gets unruly when worn more than three inches long. If you have curly, coarse hair, stay away from perfectly round helmet-shaped haircuts. They tend to look too perfect and lack movement.

Your Hair Condition: How It Affects Your Cut

The better the condition, the better the look of the cut. You can get a great haircut, but if the hair itself is overprocessed or dried out, you won't get the full benefit of the cut. Your hair cutter can recommend conditioners that will greatly improve the look of your cut.

Making the Most of the Amount of Hair You Have

● *The trick to looking good with thin hair is to keep it short.* Short hair looks fuller. A layered haircut—in which sections of hair are cut to different lengths to build bulk into the style—is a good bet. Layered hair will create fullness on the sides of your head and bulk on top, so it doesn't look flat.

● *Medium thick hair can fool you.* Some days you wake up and your hair looks luxuriously full, then again you can come home from the gym or a day at the beach and it looks like you have lost half your hair. But medium hair allows you the most versatility. The right haircut can make it look thinner or thicker. For a smoother look, get a layered cut with blunt ends. The stylist will cut sections of hair straight across, so they lie flat. For a fuller look, you'll need a layered cut using a technique called spiking, in which a stylist cuts underlying sections of the hair shorter to prop up any hair combed over it for a fuller look.

● *Having lots of hair is one of your greatest physical assets.* While any man can have great-looking hair, you don't have to work so hard. But thick hair is a treasure that can easily be squandered if it's not handled right.

If you have lots of thin-textured hair, you may not be aware of your good fortune. Because each hair shaft is narrow, your hair may not have enough texture to hold a fuller shape. It may seem to lack lift, lying flat on the head almost as soon as it emerges from the scalp. The trick to getting a great cut is to cope with this lack of lift. I usually like this kind of hair layered to add bulk in a medium length (like John DeLorean's hair). This will give the most versatility, allowing the cutter to shape the hair on the sides, top front, and back of the head according to your facial features. Thick, thin-textured hair worn long tends to swing when a man moves his head. Like Bruce Jenner, you can wear a longer, layered style for an energetic, sporty casual look.

Lots of medium-textured hair can do anything you want it to. Put it to work to bring out your face shape and best features.

Lots of coarse hair should be thinned out for more space between the hair shafts and thus more movement. Otherwise it can look like a wig (e.g., newsman Ted Koppel's hair).

Finding the Cut That Works with Your Hair Formation

Straight hair. This type hair needs to be cut in a definite shape to look good. Your stylist can create a natural, healthy look by spiking some of the hair so that when combed it has texture and movement.

Straight hair gives you many styling options:

- The back hair can be short to show off your neck and shoulders.
- The front hair can be longer, covering an overly wide forehead.
- The side hair can be cut full to narrow the face or trimmed close to the head to give the illusion of more width.

With straight hair, you can play with the proportions, stretching here and there (a little longer in back, for example) to get the job done.

Wavy hair. Depending on whether or not you like having wavy hair, decide whether you want your hairstyle to minimize or accentuate the waves. You may have wavy hair on certain parts of your head. In this case you may want either to blow-dry the wavy hair straight or get a permanent wave to unify the formation.

Curly hair. Curly hair has tremendous lift, but this can be too much of a good thing, especially if hair is cut in a bowl shape.

Because of its bulk, growing curly hair to the proper length is tricky. Grown too long (past the ears and shirt collar), curly hair begins to soften the face too much, giving a bland look. You have to judge how strong your facial features are when determining what length your curly hair should be. Curly hair is best worn short to medium length.

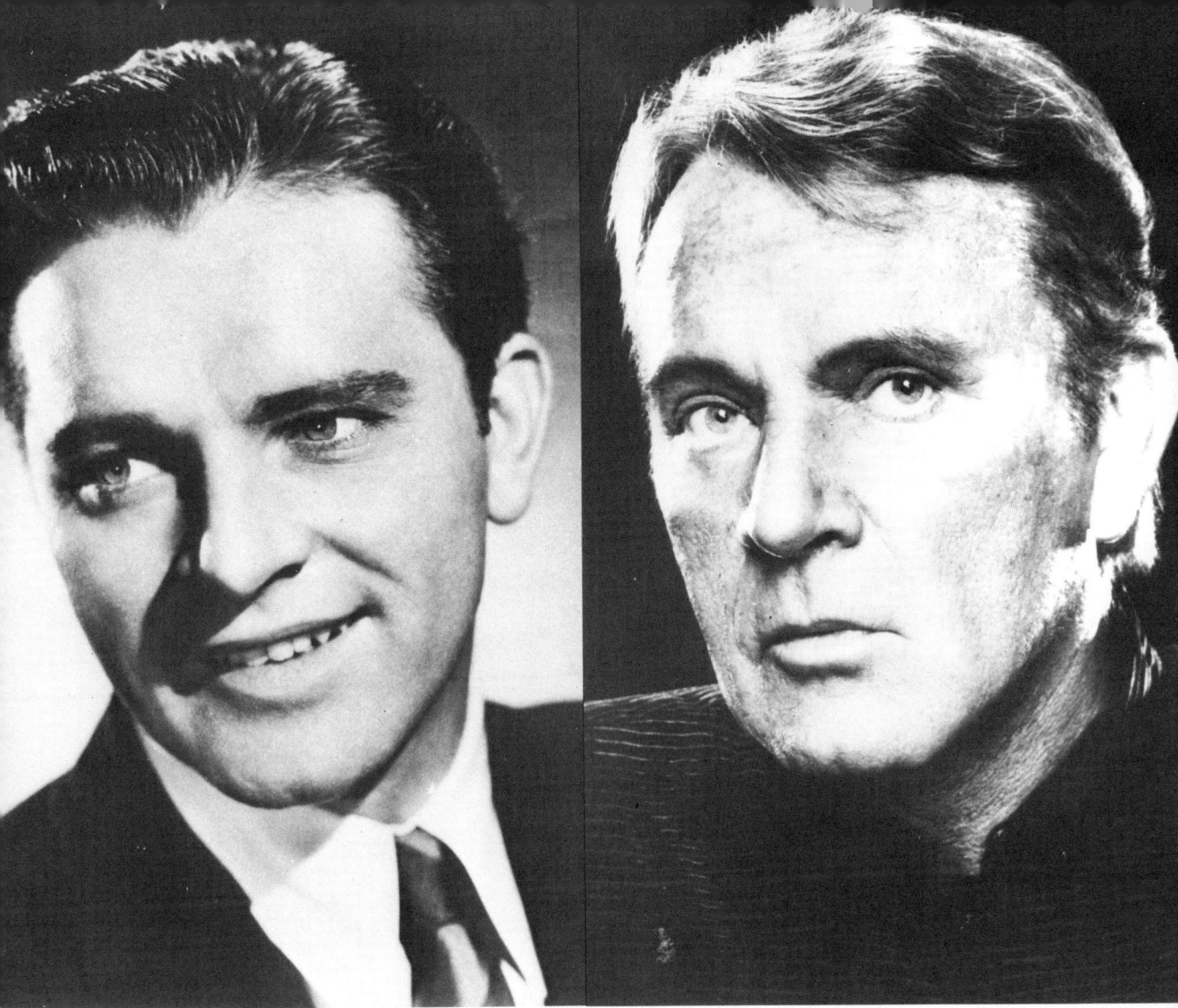

Adjusting your hair with the times

Richard Burton aged beautifully. His slick, dark hairstyle was softened as he grew older. Soft wisps of hair on his forehead and a lighter color minimize his thinning hair. The lighter hair looks thicker. Extra length in back plays up his jawline and mouth. Short hair on the sides has always given his eyes impact.

103

Facial Features

	What to Play Up	Your Options
EYES	Big eyes Long/dark lashes Strong color	Tousle on forehead to "point" at eyes Shorter hair to expose more face
EYEBROWS	Strong brow bone Thick eyebrows Dark eyebrows	Wear moustache to create balance Wear off-the-face style to expose brows
FOREHEAD	Great hairline Proportionate size	Wear hair back off the face
NOSE	Nose with character	Short hair to show off face.
EARS	Nice shape Not protruding	Totally exposed ears
MOUTH	Sensuous lips Good teeth Nice smile	Clean-shaven face
JAWLINE	Strong jaw	Clean-shaven face

What to Play Down	Your Options
Small eyes Eyes too close together	Part your hair closer to temples to "open up" forehead (makes eyes look bigger)
Wispy brows Lightly colored brows	Darken color to add impact Wear tousle on forehead to make eyes more important
Too high Too low Too wide Too narrow	Tousle to break space Hair back to enlarge space Part hair closer to center Part hair closer to temples
Too long Too short	Height on the top of the head or tousle on forehead to attract attention up Moustache to "anchor" face or short hair to make face seem larger
Large or protruding	One half inch of hair covering the top of the ear Thicker hair behind ears
Narrow lips	Moustache to strengthen mouth appearance
Weak jaw Double chin	Short beard to give squarer shape to jaw Longer hair in back to fill in neck/jaw area

Where to Part Your Hair

Seventy-five percent of all men wear some kind of part in their hair. Where should it go?

One theory is to part it where it parts naturally. To find this natural part, shake your wet hair. A part will fall into the hair. This is your natural part. Nothing says you have to comply with nature if this is not the part that looks best on you. If you do, however, your style will fall into place without a lot of help from groomers and blow dryers. I don't recommend the center part, because it calls attention to the fact that one side of your face is very different from the other.

You can use your part to help your face shape and to call attention to your eyes. The closer to the center of your head that you wear your part, the narrower your forehead will look. The farther from the center, the wider your forehead appears.

If you have a narrow face, line up your part with the outside of your eyebrow, running straight back or angled from near the center of your crown toward the outside of your eyebrow. This will visually widen your forehead. If your face is round or full, move the part closer to the center (again, never the direct center). You will notice how this slims your face immediately.

The Two Basic Haircut Shapes

All the different shapes a man's hair can have are really variations on two basic themes.

The first is a *square cut*. The hair is cut short on the sides of the head. (The sides of most men's heads are flat, so cutting the hair short on the sides gives the head a square look.) You will appear stronger, more traditionally masculine. A square cut will play up your eyes, the bone structure of your face, and your ears. The square cut works well for eighty percent of all men.

The other basic shape is the *round cut.* It is longer over the ears, covering at least half of them, with bulk on the sides. A round cut adds width to the face, especially in the temples and on the sides of the face. It's great for men with slim faces and for men who need help filling in the lower portion of the face. (The hair behind the ears should be grown thicker and longer—about one to two inches below the ears.)

Use Your Ears

A tip for getting the best look for your face, no matter what your face shape: Expose some of your ears. Leaving some ear uncovered (at least leaving the earlobes bare) draws attention to the cheekbones.

If you have large ears, you can camouflage them by growing the hair thicker behind the ear, filling in the space between the side of the head and the ear.

Barbers vs. Hair Stylists: Getting the Right Person for the Job

The main difference between barbers and stylists is their technical training. Barbers cut, but a stylist has learned everything there is to know about hair, including the techniques involved in such processes as permanents and hair coloring.

As a rule, hair stylists are more fashion-oriented. They are the equivalent of clothing designers, using hair instead of cloth to interpret the current trend. Hair stylists create the images we see on television shows, commercials, magazine layouts, films. A hair stylist will keep your look current.

Barbers are trained to be technically precise and to dole out even haircuts. They tend to mold your hair into a standard shape. Most barbers do not deal with involved hair processes like coloring and permanents.

There's a hair cutter on every block, but the person you want to handle your hair is the one who will put forth some time and creative effort. Don't be drawn to a hair cutter because of a fancy name or the great photograph in the window.

The only way to start your search for a good hair stylist is by seeking out recommendations. Look at your friends' hair. If any of them have haircuts that seem perfectly suited to their faces and personalities, if they always look well groomed, even at the beach, ask them who cuts their hair.

Ask men with great-looking hair where they get it cut. You might see someone on the street, in your office, in an elevator, *anywhere!*

There is something else to keep in mind when searching for a stylist. While you want someone with talent, you also want someone who will listen to your thoughts about the image you want to project.

How to Work with a Hair Stylist or Barber

You have scheduled an appointment with a hair stylist or barber. How can you make sure you will get the haircut you want? There are certain ground rules that make working with hair cutters easier, as

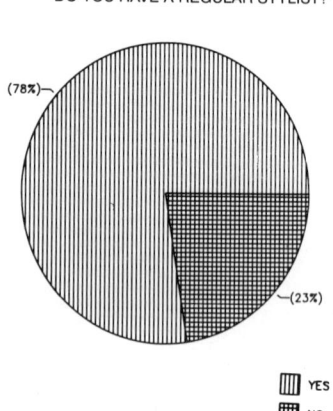

DO YOU HAVE A REGULAR STYLIST?

(78%)

(23%)

▦ YES
▦ NO

well as a vocabulary you need to know in order to communicate clearly.

The Ground Rules

First, some guidelines to get your relationship with your hair stylist off to a good start:

● **1.** Make sure the hair stylist sees you as you like to dress. If you dress like a Wall Street investment analyst during the week and would like your hair to reinforce this business like image, don't show up at the salon in casual weekend wear. The hair stylist won't see the look you want to project.

● **2.** If you are visiting a salon for the first time, talk to the hair cutter about what kind of style you would like to have *before* you change into a smock and before your hair is shampooed. Once you are in a smock with wet hair, you lose your everyday image.

If you have to rely only on verbal communication to tell the hair stylist how you ordinarily dress, you are taking a big risk.

● **3.** In most of the better hair cutting salons, it is possible to have a consultation with a hair stylist before your hair cutting appointment. This is a five- to ten-minute visit in which the stylist assesses the client's appearance and needs.

The advance consultation may give you several options to think about if you are unsure of exactly what cut you want. A good stylist will instantly visualize several hairstyles that will make you look better. For example, if a man comes to me with longer hair, I'll ask him if he wants to keep it long. If he says yes, I will imagine two or three different hairstyles in longer lengths that I think would play up his best features.

If the man says he wants to clean up his act with

I became Leonard Bernstein's hair stylist on a recommendation from his assistant, who was a friend of one of my clients. The assistant always admired my client's hair, and when Leonard complained that he couldn't get a decent haircut in New York (he was used to having his hair cut in Vienna), his assistant mentioned me, and I was called over to the maestro's apartment to cut his hair.

Most people think of Leonard Bernstein as having thick, wavy hair. So did I. But when I met him, I was surprised to discover that he actually has baby-fine hair. It is kept scrupulously clean and conditioned. The point: Even baby-fine hair can look full and dramatic if kept trimmed, conditioned, and freshly shampooed.

a shorter cut, I'll see possibilities for shorter looks. Hearing my suggestions at a consultation allows a client to go home and think about the options I've outlined, relating them to his own ideas.

You don't have to find a salon that offers consultations as part of their service. Once you have a hair cutter in mind, call him up and ask if it would be possible to speak with him for five minutes about your hair. If he is too busy to spend five minutes with you, then you probably would be better off with someone else.

Good Communications

Most poor haircuts happen because of a lack of communication. Chances are, the hair stylist wanted to give you the look you were after but didn't understand you well enough to do so.

Here are some general guidelines about how to get your message across:

● **Bring visual aids.** Many men complain that stylists invariably cut off too much hair. To make sure this doesn't happen and to help get across your overall message, bring a photo with you to the salon. It could be a photo of you looking your best or of someone you've seen in a magazine with the cut you want. This will give your stylist an immediate reference point.

Bring this book with you if you've found a hairstyle you like on one of its pages. You could also mention an actor whose hair you like. Actors pay a great deal of attention to their hair and wear styles that project the character they are playing, whether it's the sophisticated gent (Robert Wagner) or down-to-earth good ole boy (Burt Reynolds).

The male models in men's magazines are sure to

have the latest hairstyles. The best magazines for researching current hair trends are *Gentlemen's Quarterly* and *Esquire*, but even news magazines such as *Time* and *Newsweek* can be good sources of styling ideas.

• **Go over your grooming routine.** Tell the stylist how much time and effort you're willing to devote to your hair. (If the hairdresser blow-dries your hair for twenty minutes but you only use a comb to style your hair, you'll get a much different look at home.)

Don't say you'll follow a lengthy maintenance routine if you won't. Remember, it's your look, so have the stylist adapt the haircut around your needs.

• **Discuss radical changes first.** A stylist should explain what he or she is going to do before he or she does it. And if you are thinking about making a radical change in your appearance, such as having your hair colored, you have every right to expect the stylist to show you the new look on a few locks of your hair first.

Ask for this test run if your stylist doesn't offer it. In fact, in any of your dealings with a hair stylist, you should expect to ask for what you want.

If your stylist suggests a radical change, such as giving you a wave or coloring your hair, ask him to explain the process in detail; have him tell you exactly what is in it for you.

An explanation such as "You need a body wave because your hair just doesn't have texture" isn't enough. If you are not sure you need whatever the stylist is trying to persuade you to try, tell him you'll think about it.

Reread the sections of this book about the procedure in question. This should help you make up your mind.

- **Specify the right length.** On every visit to the stylist, show him exactly what length you would like your hair to be. Don't just say "medium." Show the stylist *with your hands* exactly where on your head you would like him to cut. Everyone's "one half inch" measures differently.

- **Explain your hair's habits.** It's important to tell the stylist how your hair usually behaves. For example, if you have to use a groomer every day to tame your waves, by all means give the stylist this information.

The Right Vocabulary

One trick to getting a good hair cut is to use the right words when asking for what you want. Here is a short hair styling glossary:

Blunt cutting. Cutting the hair blunt on the ends around your head—a good technique if your hair is arrow-straight.

Cowlicks. These are unusual growth patterns in the hair. Usually the hair swirls around, sticking up from the scalp. There are two ways to handle cowlicks. One is to cut the hair short, so that when it sticks up it is integrated with the rest of the style. Or your stylist can create a style with longer hair at the cowlick; the extra weight will make the hair lie flat.

You should tell your stylist where your cowlicks are and how severe a problem they pose for you.

Diffusing or nipping. Instead of cutting your hair straight across, the stylist angles his scissors when cutting sections of hair. This makes the ends of hair shafts spring up so that they don't lie flat on the head, giving more bulk to the hairstyle.

Thinning. This technique removes bulks from a hairstyle while keeping the style's overall shape intact. A special pair of scissors called thinning shears is used to even out the proportions of the haircut. As an example, if a man has more bulk on the sides and back of his head than on top, thinning could balance the haircut to call attention away from sparse areas.

Trim. A trim is a maintenance cut that removes a half inch to an inch of hair without changing the overall shape of a style. Trimming certain sections of hair is recommended every four to six weeks.

Weight. Sometimes you should ask to have weight added to certain sections of your hair, such as when it sticks out in an unruly way. For example, the hair on the back of your head may stick out instead of curling under. (It has probably been layered too much.) The hair needs to be grown thicker, so that its extra weight will hold down the problem section.

Many men have trouble when they try to grow the hair on the sides of their head longer. "Wings," sections of hair that flip up and away from the scalp and the surrounding hair, will become a problem if the hair on the sides of the head is layered too much. More weight will keep the hair integrated with the rest of the style.

What to Expect from the First Haircut

I believe a hair stylist shold be accountable for his work. You are paying for a professional service. You should get satisfaction. However, the first haircut a stylist gives you is only an introduction, and there may be certain things about your past

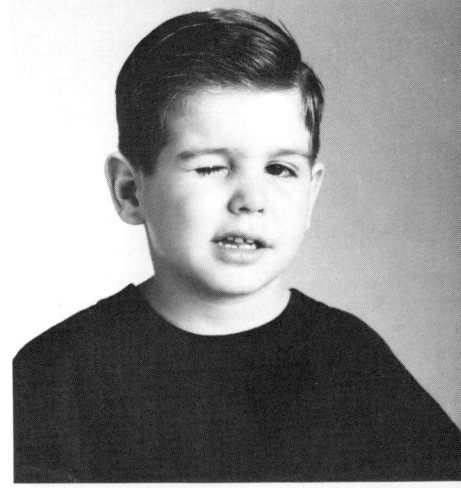

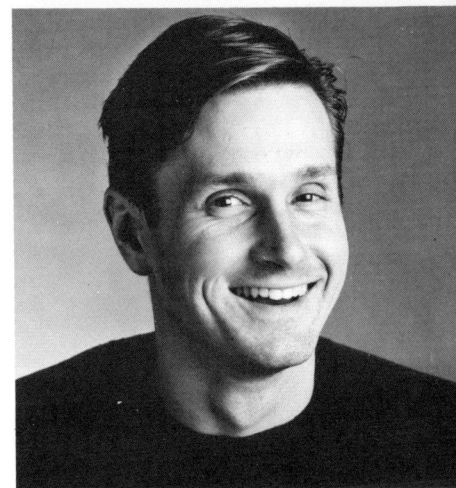

Here you see the classic military haircut. It works well for any age male. J.D., three years old, loves his. This active boy doesn't need long hair to get in his way. Mason is twenty-eight and wants maintenance-free hair. A dab of hair groomer and a finger-combing and he's out the door.

haircut that he can't correct the first time out.

For example, many men who come to me for the first time have haircuts that are proportionately out of sync. If a client's hair is too short to allow for a perfectly balanced haircut, then the only option for the stylist is to cut the hair so that by the time the client makes a second visit, his hair will be ready to accept the shape that is just right. Therefore, while your first haircut should look good, the second haircut is the one by which to judge the stylist.

The following are some tests to help you judge your haircut.

The Shake Test

Just shake your head from side to side and from front to back. Really shake it hard.

If the hair is cut well, you should be able to shape it back into style using only your fingers—no brush, no comb. Simply comb your hair with your fingers. If the hairstyle assumes a well-defined but casual-looking shape, chances are you have a good cut.

The Wet Test

Do this test when you get out of the shower. Again, shake your head and try to push your hairstyle into shape. You should be able to see a definite shape to the cut even when it's wet. The hair should fall into a flattering shape that looks right for the shape and proportion of your face.

The Edge Test

The edges of the haircut should be neat, especially on the sides and back of the head. You would think any hair cutter could give you a haircut with even lines, but it takes careful cutting to achieve well-sculpted edges.

Trimming Your Hair at Home

Many men think that they can give themselves a great home haircut or that their wives or friends can cut their hair just as well as a trained hair stylist. I can honestly say that most home haircuts I've seen have been disastrous.

While cutting your own hair is not a good idea, trimming your hair at home is a good way to keep your cut looking fresh and save some money, too.

You can help your hair look better longer and not have to go back to the hair stylist as often. The trick is to keep the amount of hair you cut to a minimum and to limit the areas where you do your trimming.

How to Trim the Front Section of Your Hair

You know it's time to trim the hair at the front of your head when

- It hangs in your eyes.
- It won't stay in place.
- It's getting too thick to manage.
- It irritates your forehead.

Start one inch in back of your hairline and comb the front of your hair forward over your forehead. Don't wet your hair. Your hair is longer when it's wet, so you may cut too much hair. Leave wet cutting to the professionals. Cutting your dry hair will be fine for a quick shape-up.

Comb the hair in front of the front section out of the way of the scissors. (You can buy some inexpensive hair clips at any drugstore to hold this hair back.)

Hold the hair at the front of your head between your index finger and your middle finger and slide

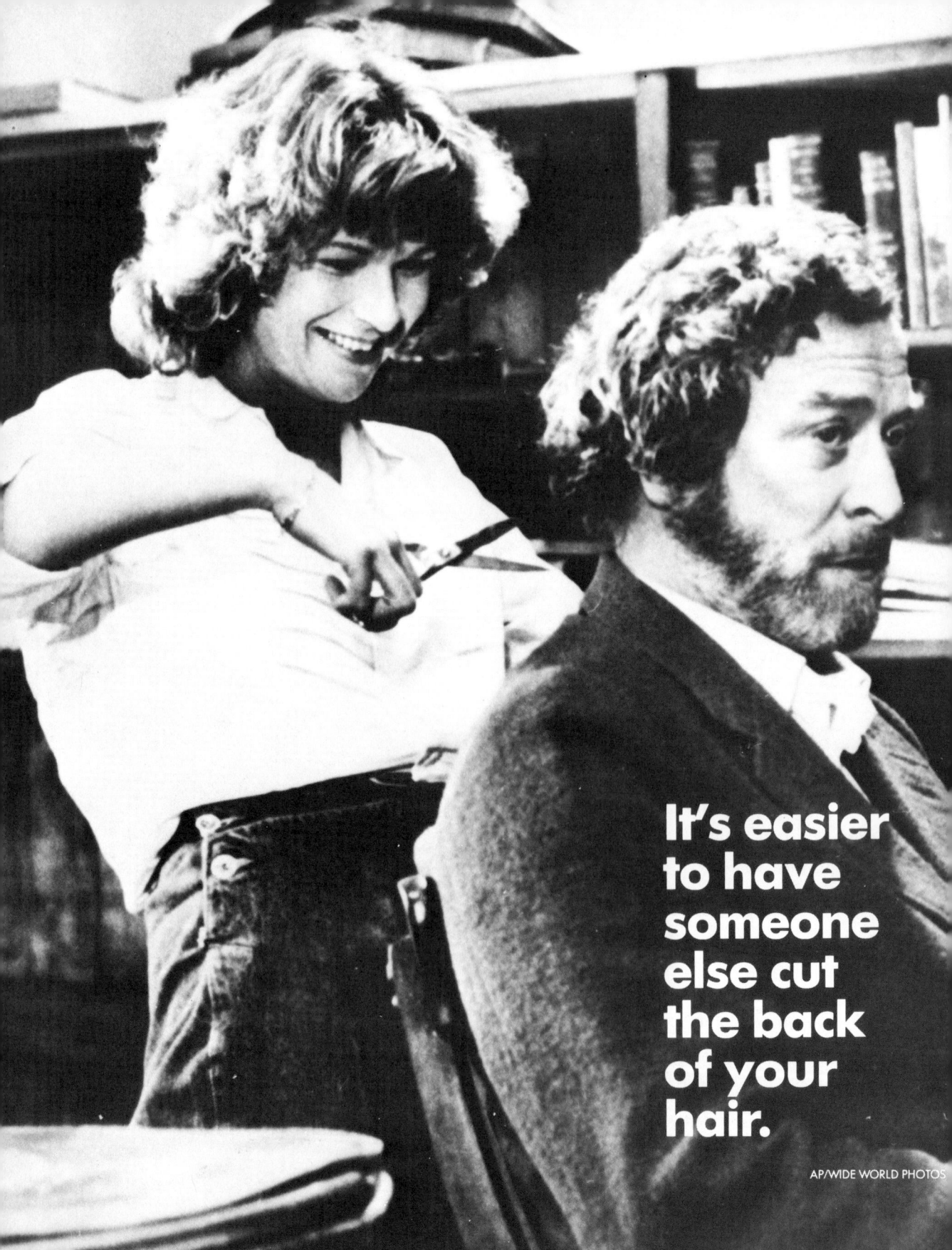

It's easier to have someone else cut the back of your hair.

your fingers down the hair to where you want to cut it.

You only want to cut hair shafts that fall between the pupils of your eyes. Cutting only the hair inside these boundaries will shorten the hair in front, while cutting outside of the pupils may interfere with the way the sides of the haircut fall.

When you cut the hair, don't cut straight across or you run the risk of looking like the lad on the Dutch Boy paint labels. Instead, hold the scissors straight up, pointing toward the ceiling. Tip them to a slight angle and cut small pie-shaped sections out of the hair hanging below your fingers. This will eliminate some length while keeping the hair natural-looking.

How to Trim the Sideburns and the Area Around the Ear

The hair growing around the ear is the first to show signs of growth after a haircut. You can keep your haircut fresh longer by trimming the lines that begin at the inside bottom corner of your sideburns and run around the ear.

If you have *short hair,*

● First comb your hair back. The hair between your sideburns and your ear will not have as well defined a line as when your hair was originally cut.

● Trim the hair between the sideburn and the ear in a straight line, and cut around the top of the ear.

● To finish the trim, bend your ear forward and hold it down while you trim the hair in back of the ear.

● Remember, this is only a trim. Cut no more than a quarter inch of hair.

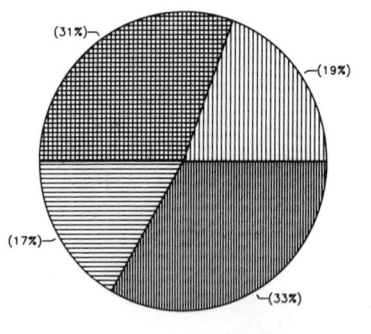

HOW LONG DO YOU GO BETWEEN HAIRCUTS?

(31%)

(19%)

(17%)

(33%)

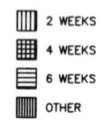

▥ 2 WEEKS
▦ 4 WEEKS
▤ 6 WEEKS
▥ OTHER

If you have *medium or long hair* (two inches or longer),

● Use the same procedure as outlined above for trimming the hair between the sideburns and your ears, but don't cut around the ear.

● To trim the hair hanging over the ears, comb the hair down over them and trim up to a half inch, following the line of the original cut. Don't make your own line!

How to Trim the Back of the Haircut

To trim the hair at the back of your head, you will need two mirrors, patience and a steady hand—or a friend who will do the job for you.

Position the mirrors so that you don't have to hold them while looking at the back of your head. If you have a short haircut with a natural hairline, don't try to trim it yourself, because the hair is too short. Instead, clip the fuzz from the back of the neck to neaten up the hairline.

If you have a shaped hairline, you should be able to trim it with no problem. Comb your hair flat against your neck and hold it down with one hand. With the other hand, use the scissors to cut off about a half inch of hair (again, following the line of the stylist).

How Long Should a Haircut Last?

Using the trimming methods outlined above, a great haircut should last six to ten weeks. The hair will grow longer, but it will not grow out of shape. If after two weeks your haircut is looking lopsided or sections of hair seem to be growing out in different directions the cut is bad.

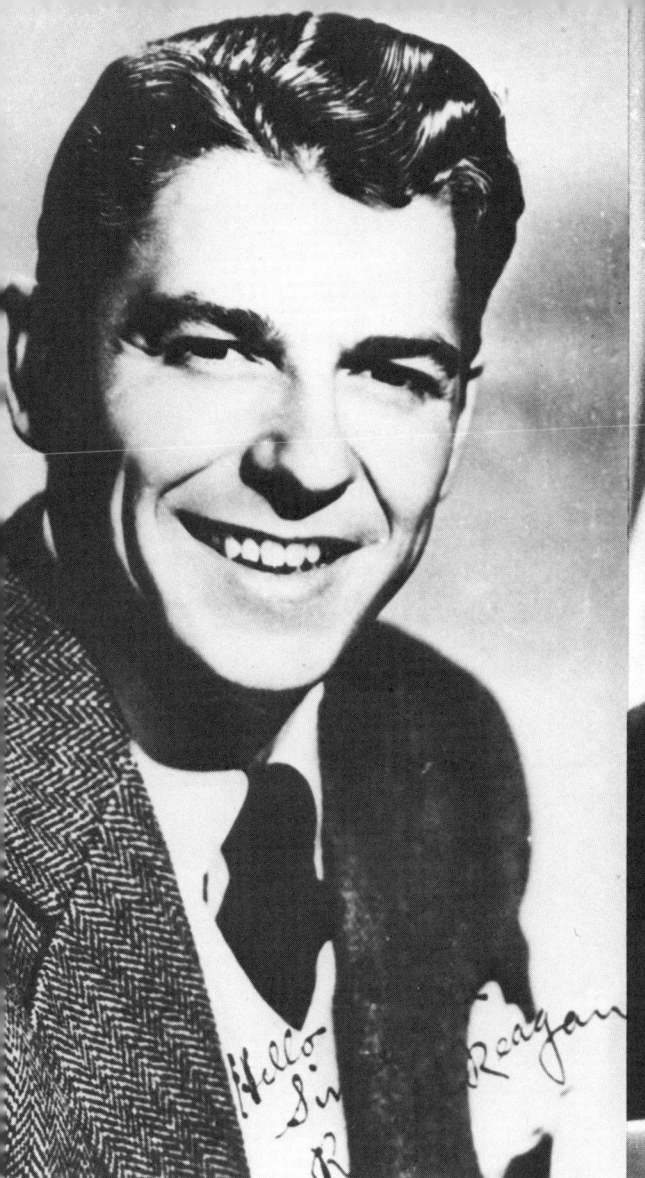

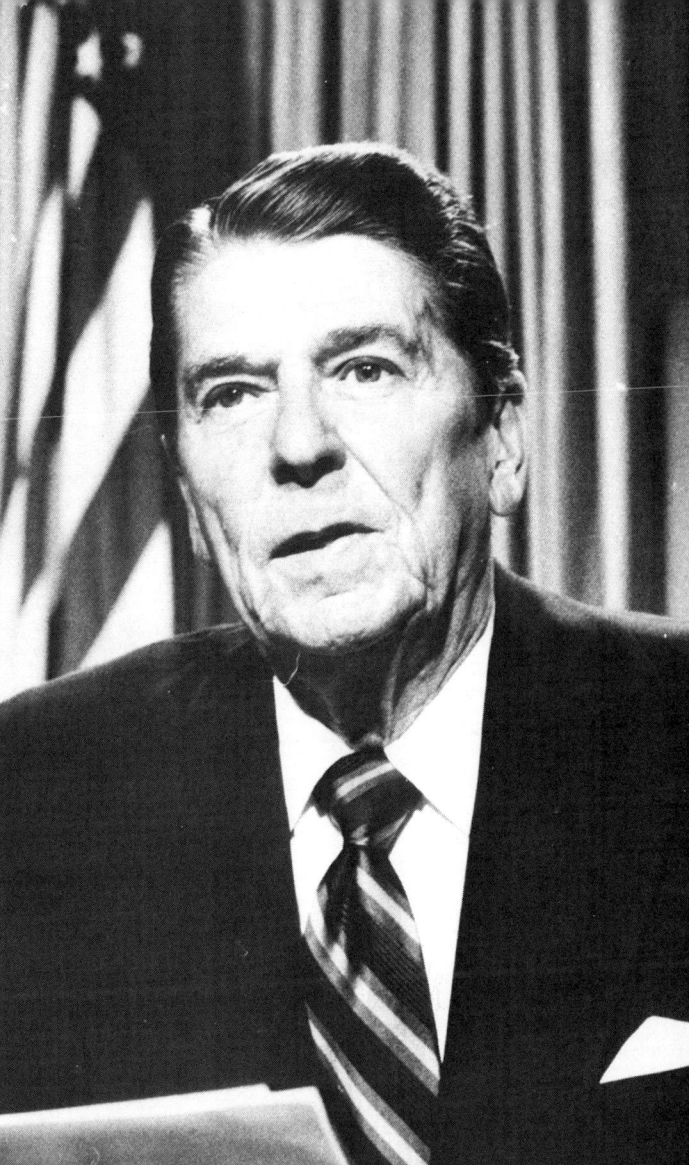

If a haircut works, stick with it!

Ronald Reagan has worn the same shape haircut for decades: side-parted to widen his forehead and short on the sides to accentuate his eyes. It works well for his face and plays up his strong hairline. It's always short enough to hold its shape and stay perfectly groomed. This particular haircut will work for any age man if he has the right hair qualities.

119

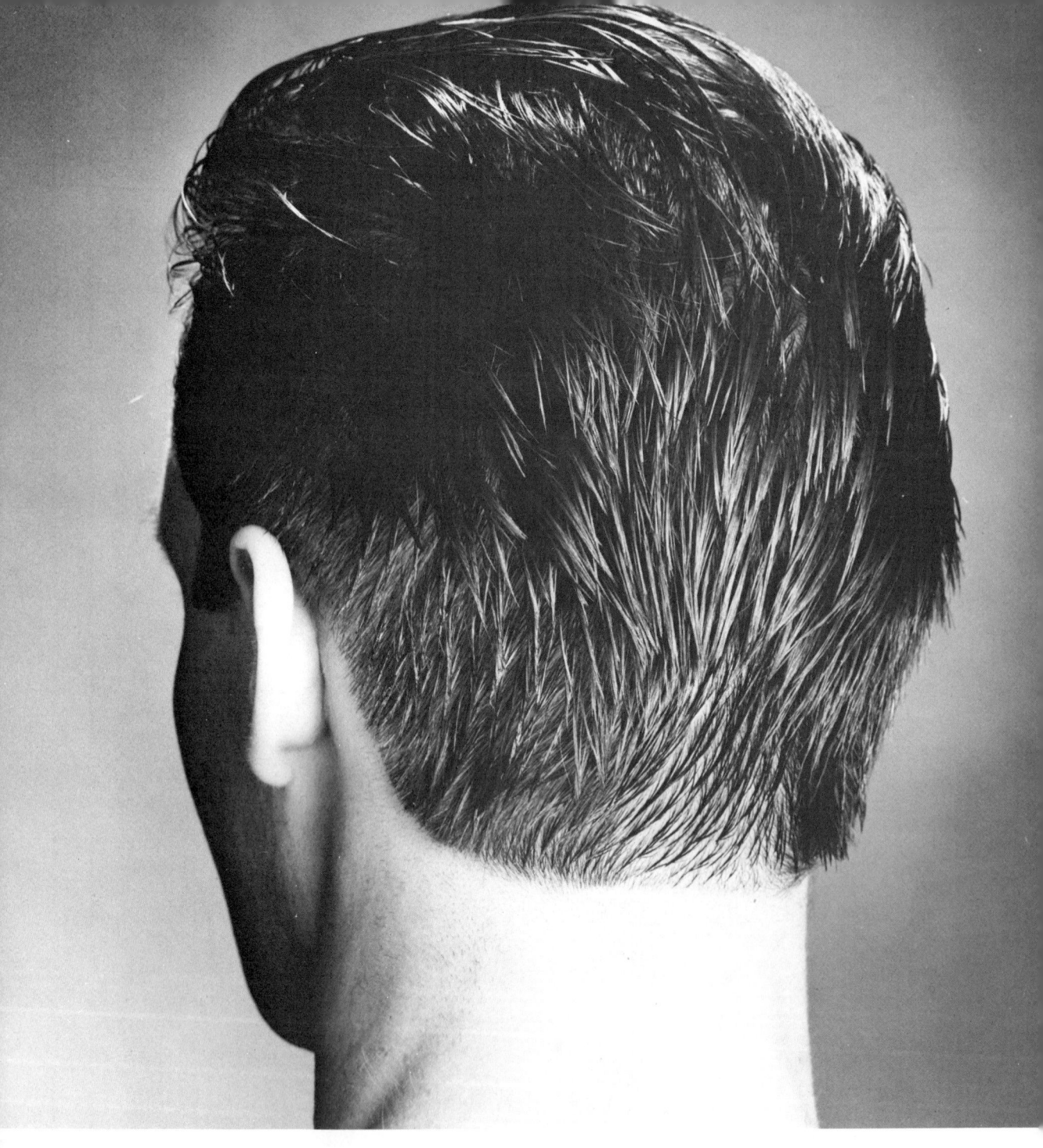

A shaped hairline
has a definite design line.

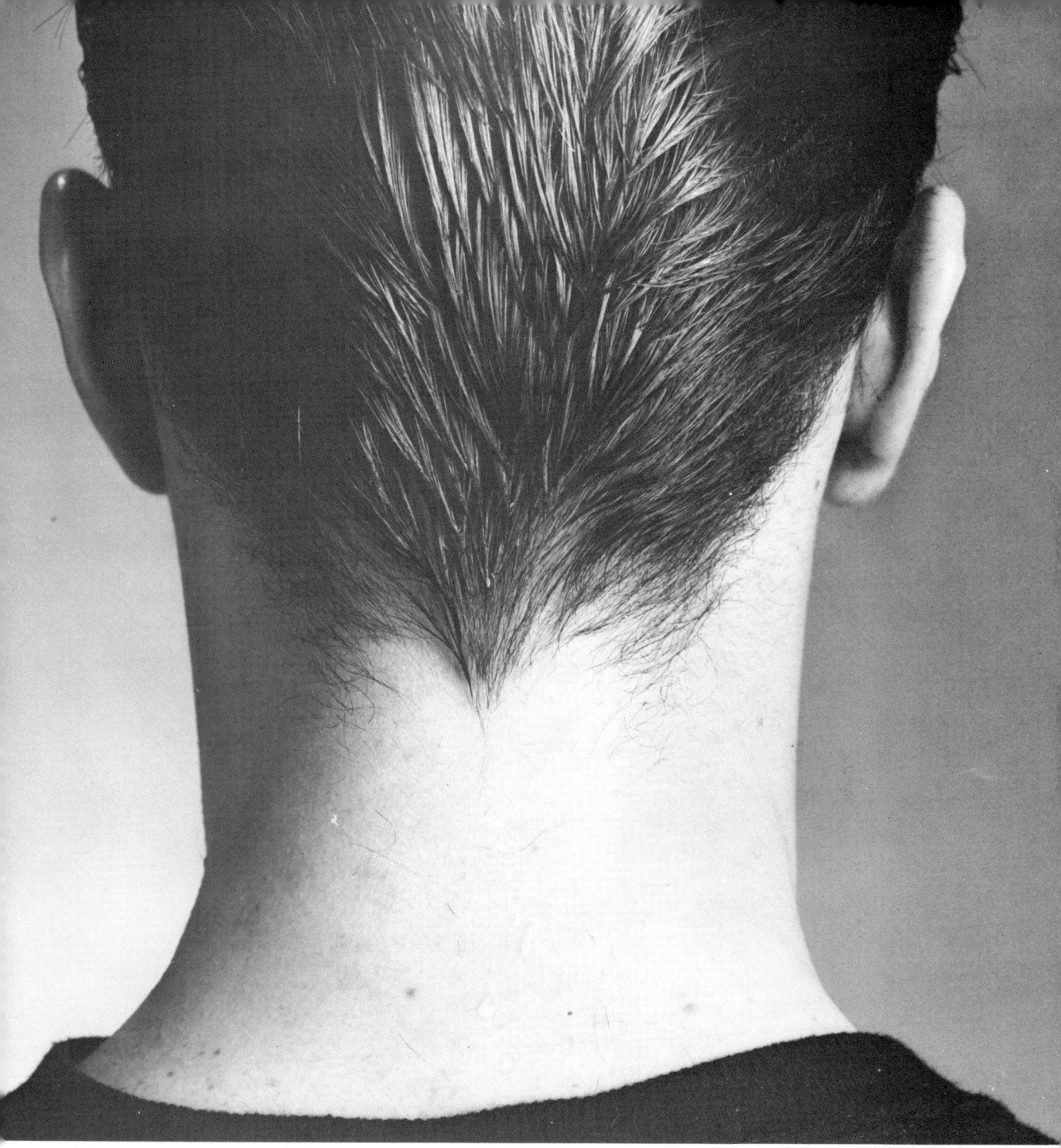

**No definite shape is
cut into a natural hairline.**

- A short cut (one half to one inch in the back) will grow out in about six weeks.
- A medium-length cut (one to three inches in back) will take about eight weeks.
- Long hair (over three inches in back) will last ten weeks.

How Much Should a Haircut Cost (and Is It Worth Paying More)?

The cost of a haircut has little to do with its quality. For example, in New York City, you can spend anywhere from $3 to $300 for a haircut, with the majority of good stylists working for a fee somewhere in between.

At the top salons you should expect to pay anywhere from $20 to $60. Is it worth the price? I believe it's worth whatever you have to pay to get the cut you need. If you're wearing a $500 suit but your hair isn't right, what good does the suit do?

If you can find a hair stylist who does wonderful work for a low fee, then by all means use him. If not, spring for the extra money and be satisfied.

Tipping

Here are some rules on how to tip.

- If the person who cuts your hair owns the salon, it's proper not to tip.
- If the stylist works for the salon, a tip of fifteen to twenty percent is proper.
- If someone shampoos your hair, you should tip them a dollar.
- If the stylist has an assistant who helps you, he or she also should be tipped a dollar or two.

6

MAINTENANCE

A Good Haircut Should Demand Minimal Daily Care

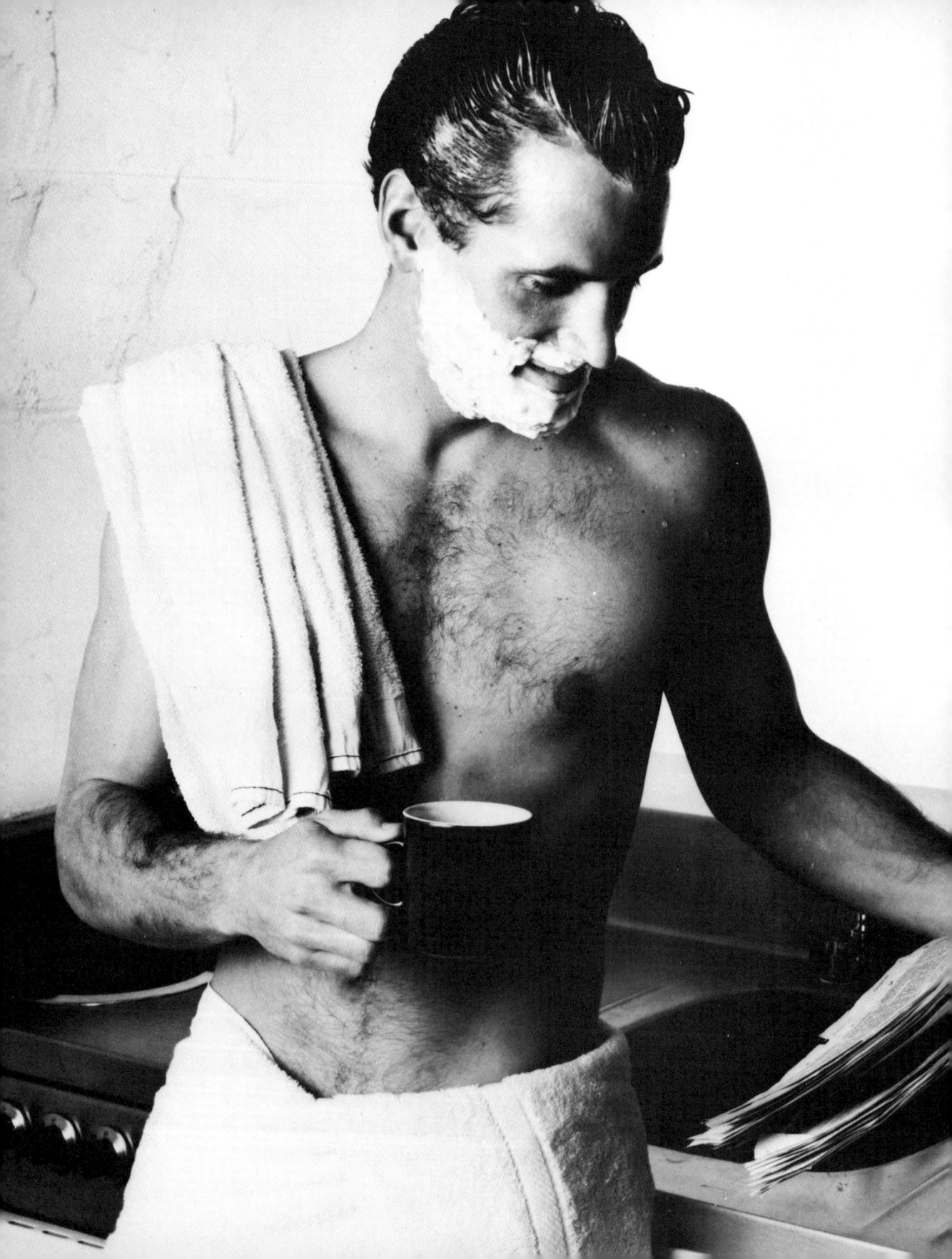

Keeping Your Hair Looking Its Best

Once you leave the hair stylist, it's up to you to keep your hair good-looking and well groomed. If you have a good haircut and your hair is in good condition, it should virtually fall into shape with a minimum of effort. All you need is the right shampoo and finishing rinse, a conditioner to protect your hair, and perhaps a groomer. Your maintenance routine should be uncomplicated, easy to do, and most important, right for you.

Shampoos and Shampooing

What You Need to Know about Shampoos

If you're used to shampooing with *anything* that lathers, you're not treating your hair right. Body soap, for instance, is far too alkaline. It's drying to your hair and leaves a dull film. Though any shampoo will get your hair reasonably clean, some will do more for your particular type of hair than others. It is difficult to sort through the fads and hype of the shampoo business—herbals one minute, protein shampoos the next—to pick your best bet. You can't go wrong, however, picking according to your hair type.

Oily Hair. Oily hair poses a particular shampoo problem. It needs thorough cleaning to remove oil from the scalp, but you shouldn't use creamy shampoos. They leave a coating on your hair that you don't need. If you shampoo often, the strong

125

cleansing shampoos designed for oily hair may be too hard on your hair in the long run. Stick to a shampoo formulated for normal hair types. Or try Clinique shampoo—it has no additives to weigh the hair down.

Normal Hair. Normal hair has fewer oil glands, so it does not need to be shampooed as often as oily hair. A moderately creamy shampoo is best, because it will not only clean the hair but add a bit of moisture to the hair shafts. Fermodyl makes several types of moderately creamy shampoo.

Dry Hair. Dry hair has the fewest oil glands. It needs to get and retain as much moisture as possible, and it must have very gentle treatment. You probably won't have to shampoo it as frequently—

Matching your shampoo to your hair's needs improves its shine and texture. Proper conditioning will strengthen and soften your hair. Use a finishing rinse daily to protect and tame your hair.

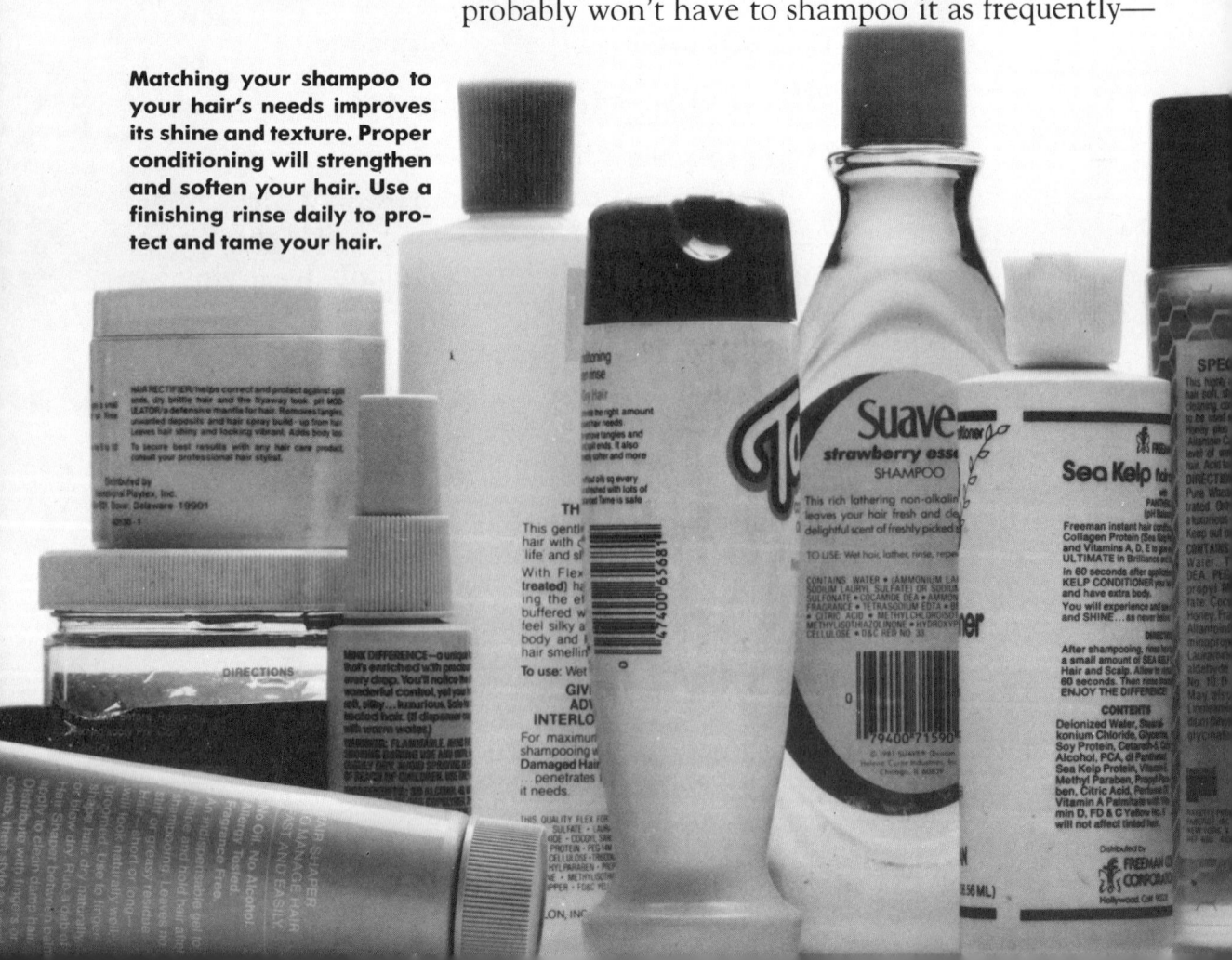

getting your hair squeaky clean means you're robbing too much moisture from it. Look for creamy shampoos or those marked for dry, damaged hair. They are the kindest to your type of hair. Pantene's shampoo for color-treated hair is a good choice for you.

Why You May Need a Variety of Shampoos

Sometimes your shampoo may seem to stop working after a while. That's because your hair and scalp change from day to day. Though your hair is dead, a waste product of the body, it can get drier and more porous through exposure to the elements, or more oily if your scalp becomes more oily through a change in diet or body chemistry.

If your favorite shampoo seems to be giving up,

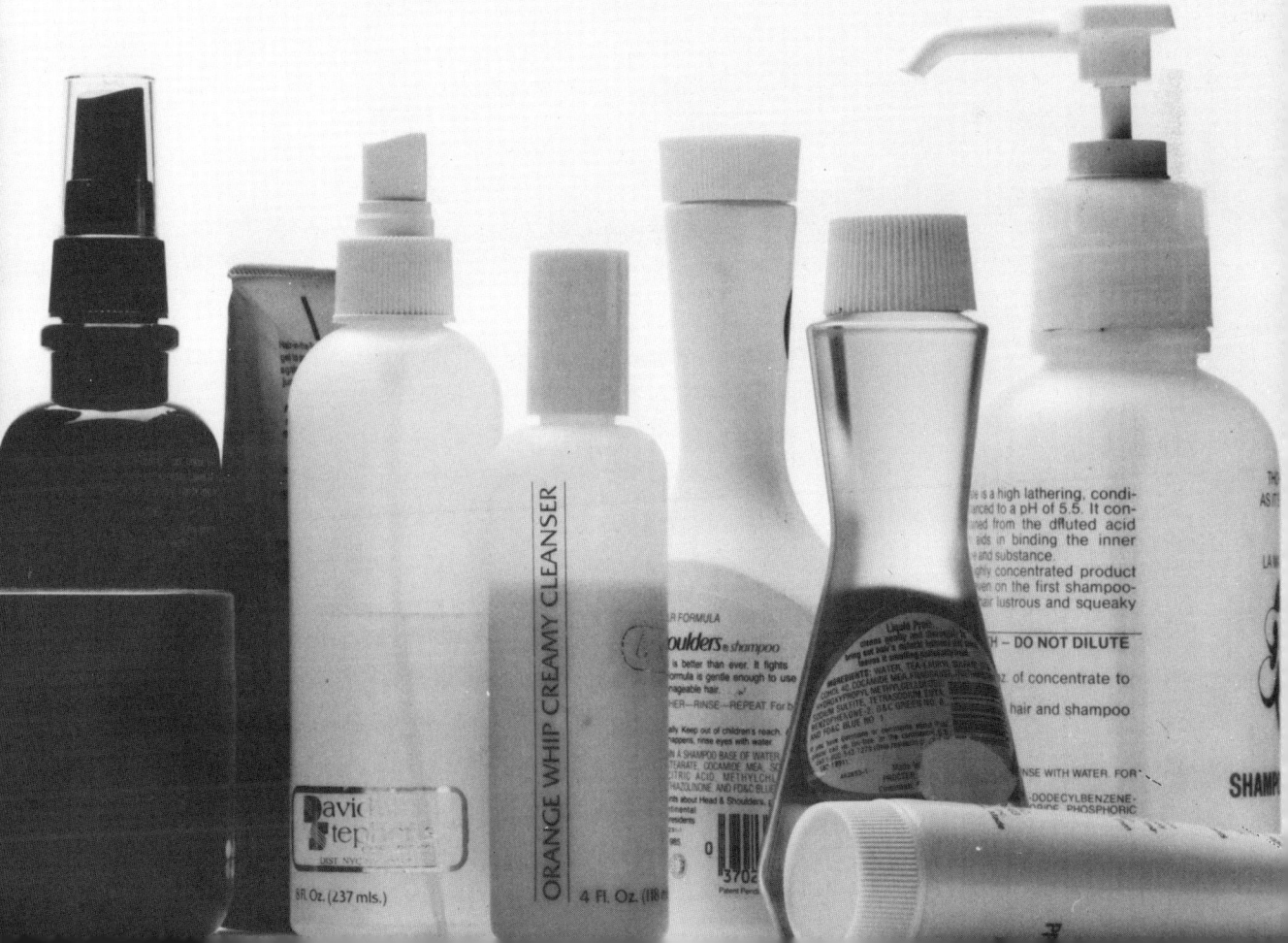

(74%)

(18%)

(8%)

DAILY
>DAILY
NON-DAILY

switch to another type for a while. It's a good idea to keep two or three different shampoos on hand and vary their use from day to day.

How Often to Shampoo

Besides shampooing when your hair looks dirty, there are some other considerations:

- **Your hair type.** Oily hair can be shampooed once or twice daily. Dry hair can go the longest; it really only needs to be shampooed three times a week.
- **The climate.** Your body produces more oil in warmer weather. You'll need to shampoo more often in summer than in winter.
- **Exercise.** If you exercise often, you speed up oil production. You should shampoo after your workout. If you exercise in the afternoon or evening, just rinse your hair in the morning and save the shampoo for later. But don't get caught in the trap of shampooing too often; you'll dry the hair shafts.

What Happens When You Shampoo

When you shampoo, you remove residue from the hair and scalp. Smoke, dust, hair groomers—all are washed away. You also remove protective oils. But you can't fool Mother Nature. As soon as you finish cleaning the scalp, your body starts working to replace the oil you've just lost.

Therefore, the more often you shampoo, the more often you'll need to shampoo. If you'd like to shampoo less often, you will have to get your scalp in the habit of producing less oil. Try shampooing every other day for a while. Your hair may look too oily for a week or so, then amazingly it will adjust itself to your new routine.

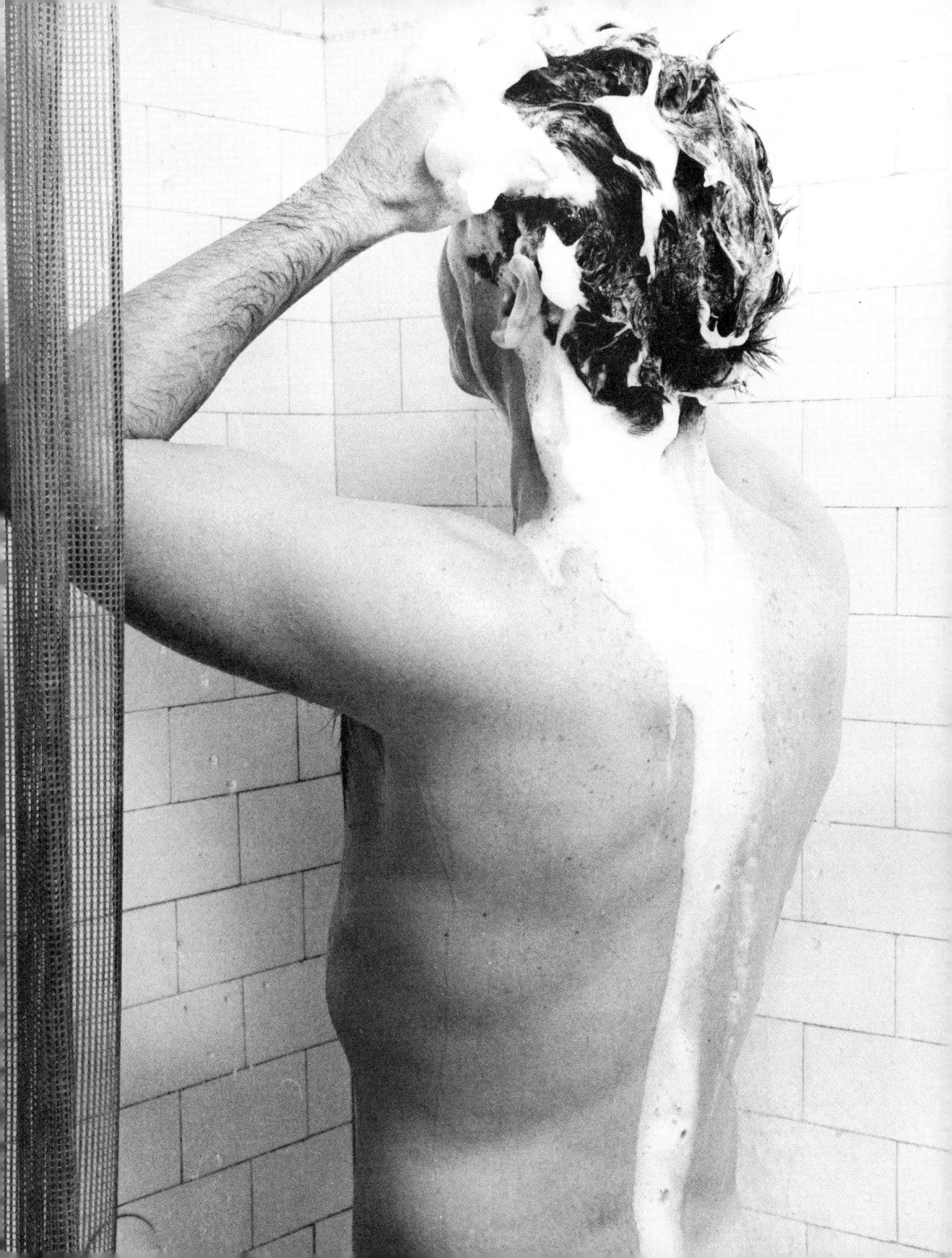

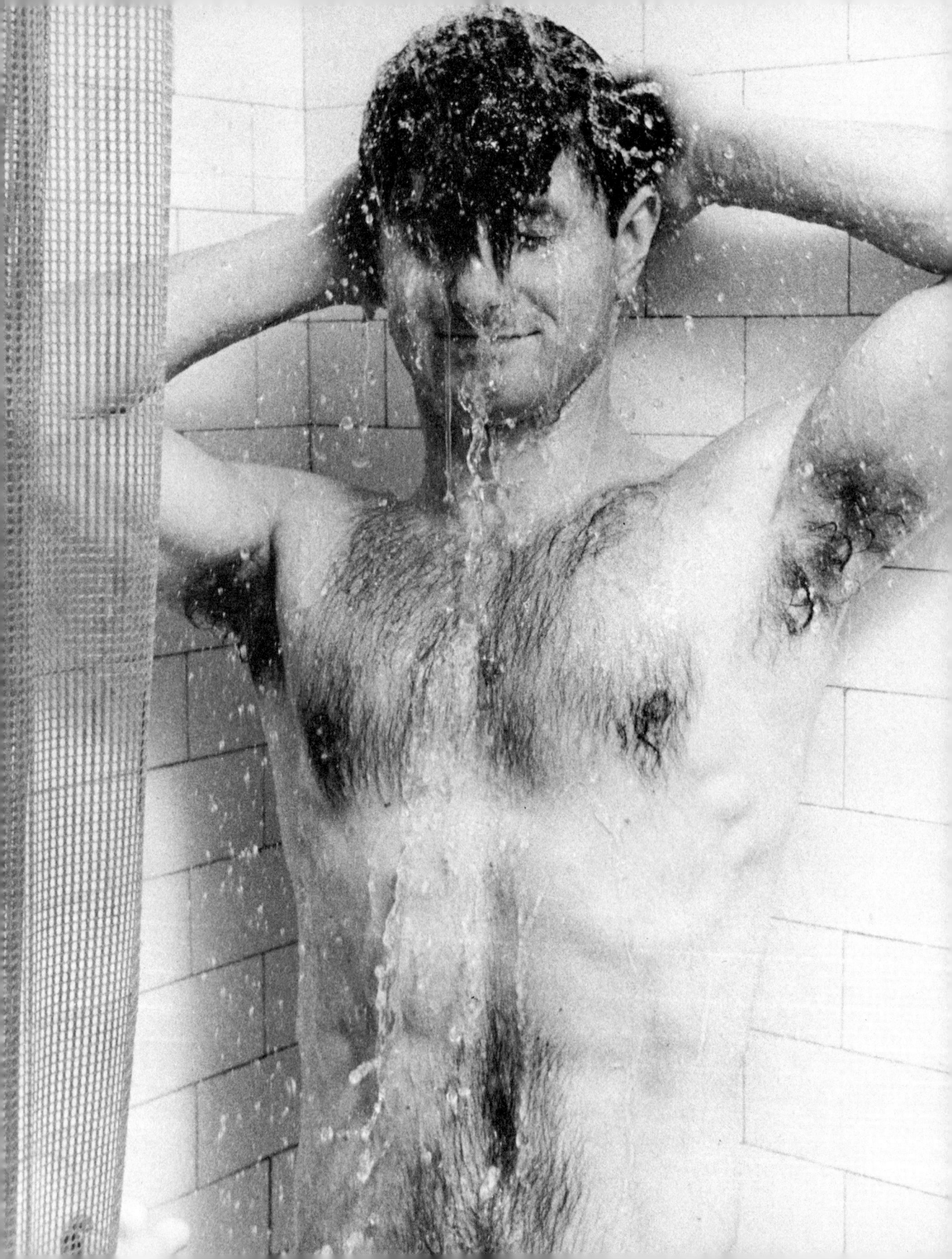

The Right Way to Shampoo

First bend from the waist and give your hair a good brushing (scalp included) with a combination nylon/natural bristle brush. Brush with upward strokes to stimulate the blood supply to the scalp and to feed the hair follicles. This also loosens any scalp flakes that need to come off.

In the shower, start with a good soaking with comfortably cool water—the cooler the water, the better. Cooler water cuts through the shampoo and oils best and helps smooth down the cuticle of the hair for extra shine.

Next, pour a quarter-sized dollop of shampoo into your palm and rub your hands together to distribute it evenly. With slightly open fingers, begin to massage your scalp using the pads of the fingers (not the nails—they might scratch the scalp). Start at your temples and work your way to the top of the head. Then start at the nape of your neck and work your way up the back.

Your hair will be cleaned as the shampoo slides along the hair shafts. You don't need to scrub your hair! Follow with a rinse of water, then rinse again. Make sure to get all the shampoo out of your hair. Often men think they have dandruff when they really have shampoo left in their hair that flakes out when it dries. It can also clog scalp pores and oil glands. So good, thorough rinsing is very important. (One lathering, however, is enough. Two latherings will only dry out the hair shaft—and sell more shampoo.)

The Finishing Rinse: What It Does

A finishing rinse is a product that you can put on the hair after you shampoo. It does several things.

- *It detangles.*

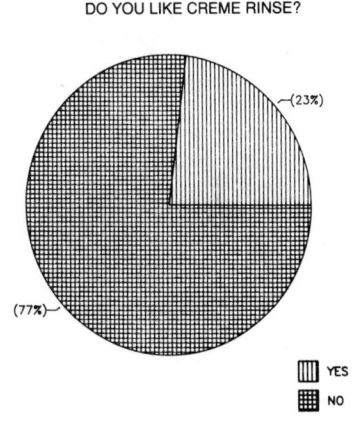

DO YOU LIKE CREME RINSE?

(23%)

(77%)

|||| YES
||||| NO

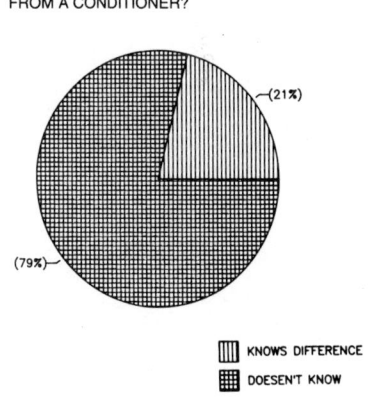

IS A CREME RINSE DIFFERENT FROM A CONDITIONER?

(21%)

(79%)

|||| KNOWS DIFFERENCE
||||| DOESEN'T KNOW

131

- *It protects the hair by leaving a slight coating.*
- *It cuts down on static, especially in winter.*
- *It adds shine.*
- *It adds manageability.*

A finishing rinse will smooth down the hair shaft with a lighter coating than that provided by a creme rinse. It's good for taming and laying down thick, bushy flyaway hair. But it won't help fine hair that needs lift and body.

I've found the best finishing rinse to be ACV Plus, by Mahdeen Laboratories. It's good for most hair types, never greasy or heavy. Klorane products are also excellent. For curly and wavy hair, try Flex finishing rinse. It's heavier than the others, thus good for calming down frizzy hair.

Conditioners and Conditioning

The Difference Between a Finishing Rinse and a Conditioner

A finishing rinse simply finishes a shampoo. You leave it on for only a minute.

A conditioner is left on the hair from three minutes to an hour. It acts as a moisturizer for the hair and needs to penetrate the hair shaft. If you leave your conditioner on for only two minutes, you won't be getting the full benefit of the product. Climatress, by Redken Labs, is an excellent moisturizer for the hair. You apply it to freshly shampooed hair and leave it on for at least ten minutes, then rinse out.

Why You Need a Conditioner

A conditioner puts back into hair what the hair needs. Because your hair is "dead," the oil that comes from your scalp takes a long time to reach the end of the hair shaft. The hair itself can become dried out, porous, dull, brittle.

To get your hair to look its best, you need to give it two things it has lost: moisture and protein.

- Moisture makes the hair soft, flexible, more resistant to breakage. And because the cuticle lies flatter, soft hair also shines more.

- Protein penetrates the hair. It plumps up the hair shaft and makes the hair stronger.

How Often to Condition

Depending on the damage to your hair, condition at least once a week for fifteen to thirty minutes. If you have dry, frizzy, or too-curly hair, you'll need to condition more often to repair it or to tame it. By using a conditioner three times a week, the hair will improve dramatically, look softer, healthier, and more controllable.

If your hair is in good shape, you'll only need to do the minimum of conditioning to maintain it.

Hot Oil Treatments

Although so considered by many people, hot oil treatments are not really conditioners. They do not add protein or moisture. They were used in the '50s for dry scalp treatment and remain a popular home remedy. The procedure is to apply a vegetable oil to the scalp and wrap the head with hot towels or a heating cap, then rinse out the oil. Again, this is best for dry scalp, not for hair.

Conditioning Hints

- Slather on conditioner before you go out in the sun and before you swim in a pool. It will protect your hair from drying out in the sun and damage from pool chemicals.

- Another great reason for wearing conditioner

How to Tell if Your Hair Needs Moisture

Moist hair is
- **Soft to touch**
- **Almost never frizzy**
- **Shiny**
- **Has no split ends**
- **Lies down on the head better**

Dry hair is
- **Brittle, breaking or snapping off easily, like straw**
- **Has a flat, dull light, as if it has been powdered, instead of a shiny, rich reflection**
- **Frequently has split ends**
- **Is difficult to control**

These types of hair usually need moisture: thick hair, curly hair, wavy hair, long hair, colored or permed hair.

Conditioners need a minimum of three minutes to absorb. The longer you leave them on, the better.

on your hair at the beach is that the sun's heat will help it penetrate. After the beach, just rinse your hair. It will look great, soft and shiny!

• The longer it stays on your hair, the more benefit you get from your conditioner. Why not try sleeping with it on your hair once a week?

Groomers

A groomer is anything you put into your hair to build body, add texture and shine, and help hold your hair in place.

Hair Sprays

Hair sprays have changed a great deal. They are no longer heavy, stiff, sticky lacquers. They often contain formulas with sun screens and conditioners. You can find them in nonaerosol sprays as well as aerosol. The only difference between men's and women's hair spray is the scent and packaging.

There is a correct way to use hair spray. After your hair is dry—whether dried naturally or with a blow dryer—hold the container four to six inches away and spray the top of the hair. Wait a minute and then finger-brush or vent-brush your hair. Your hair will remember the hold, and you'll avoid the plastered down, stiff hair look.

Gels. Gels are clear and greaseless. They make your hair thicker and give it staying power by coating the hair shaft with a clear film. Gels are good for anyone who wants a wet shiny look.

Gels should be applied to damp hair only. After shampooing and towel-drying your hair, put a dollop of gel the size of a fifty cent piece in the palm of your hand. Rub your hands together and, starting at the roots of your hair, apply the gel to your hair. When your hair dries, it will feel crispy and hard; it will look wet. You can leave it as is if you like the wet look or brush it with a brush or your fingers for a freer style that still retains a definite shape.

Clinique's Hair Shaper, Aramis Multiplexx, and Tenax are some good gels. Just as good, but less expensive are Dippity Do and DEP.

Mousse. A mousse, dispensed by an aerosol can, is a foam that looks like shaving cream. It's not as sticky as a gel and can be used on dry hair and longer hair.

Rub the mousse into your hair any place you want lift or body. Because the mousse is mostly air, you will need to use more than you would a gel. Start with an amount the size of an egg, dispensed in your palm. Don't rub your hands together. Just dip into the mousse with your free hand and apply to specific areas where you want more lift or control. Some good mousses are made by L'Oreal, La Coupe, and Alberto Culver.

1. Hair spray
2. Oily groomer
3. Gel
4. Mousse
5. Setting lotion
6. Water

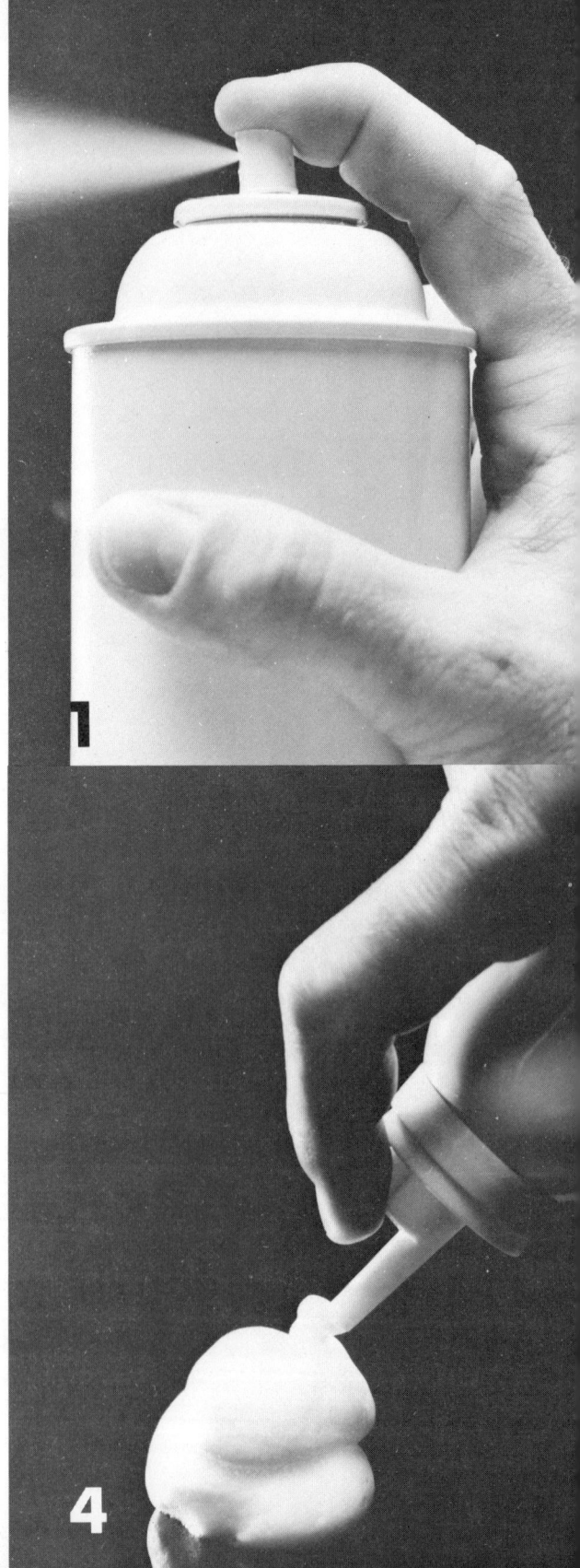

4

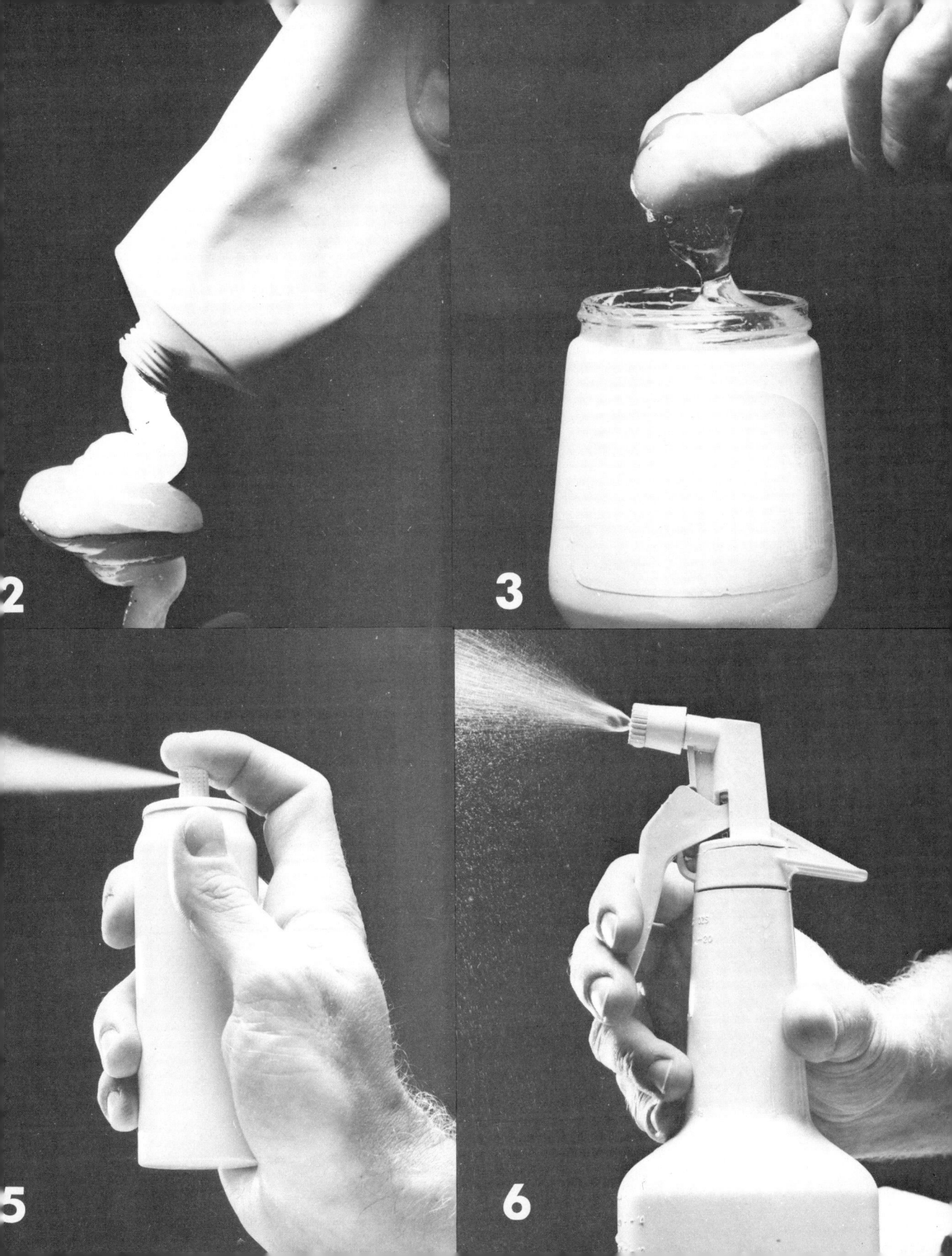

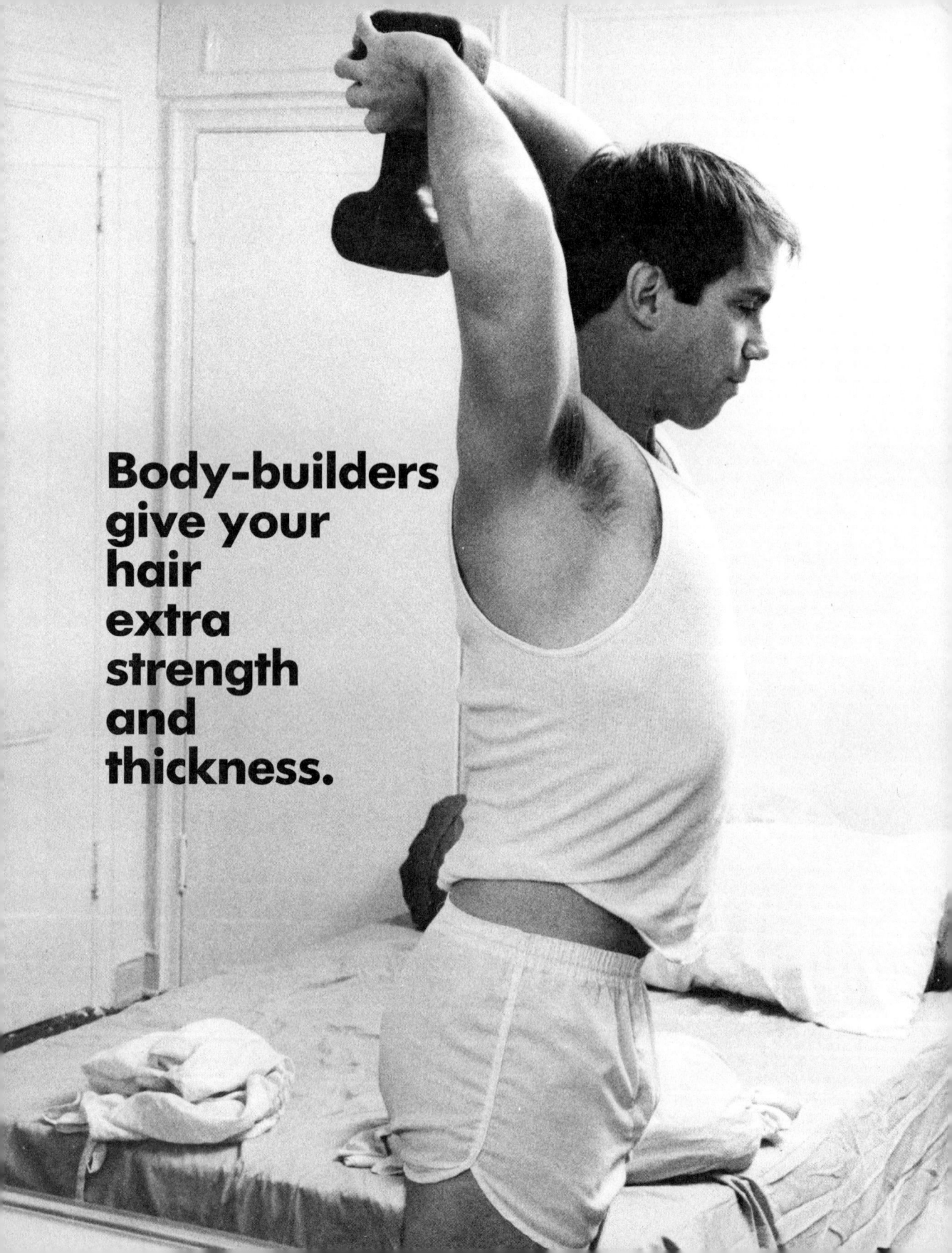

Body-builders give your hair extra strength and thickness.

Body-builders

Gel, mousse, and setting lotion are all body-builders. They coat the individual hair strands and stiffen them. Gels build the most body, giving hair the thickest coating.

Setting Lotion. Setting lotions are nonaerosol sprays. Basically they are liquid thickeners. These are best used on hair that is to be blown dry. Thicket and Pantene Setting Spray are two good ones. Spray them on damp hair, only at the roots. The lotion will then mix with the water still on your hair for a nonsticky finish.

Setting lotion gives a thick coating but less crispiness than gels. Mousses are the lightest; they give the hair body without leaving a stiff residue on the hair.

The thicker your hair, the heavier the body-builder you can wear. Thick, coarse hair could use a gel; medium hair, a setting lotion; thin, fine hair, a mousse.

If you're working with a body-builder/groomer for the first time, you have to experiment to find the right amount to use.

Body-builders and groomers can make your hair thicker and shinier than you ever imagined. When you see what they can do for your hair and your look, you'll want to make them a part of your daily grooming routine. Experiment with them all.

Sometimes if your hair is too clean, it can look too perfect. A hair groomer can then give your hair a more rumpled, casual look.

Oily Hair Groomers

These groomers come in a tube. You only need a little dab the size of a pinky fingernail. They add shine and manageability. Use them on thick-to-

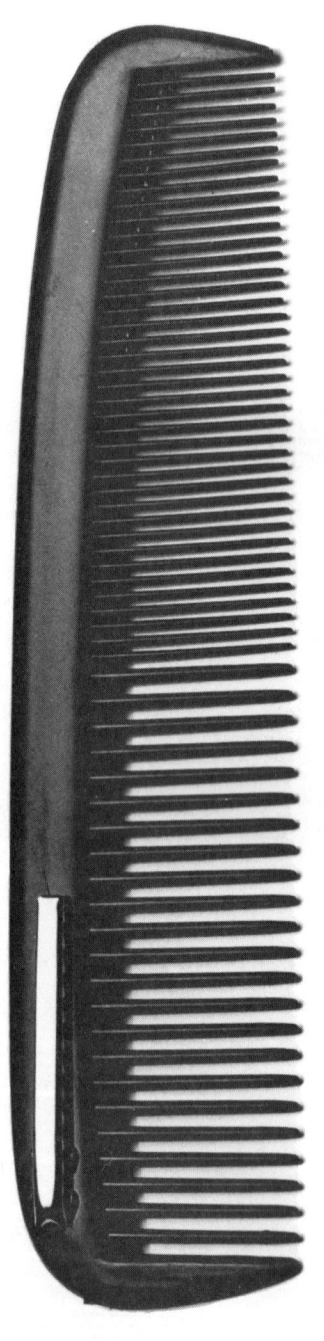

medium hair, coarse hair, or curly hair. They hold hair in place and add light reflection to dull hair. The best are Brylcreem, VO5, and Vitapoint. These can be used on wet or dry hair. Put a dab in your hand, rub your hands together, and then smooth into the hair.

Equipment

Combs

There are only two types of combs a man will ever need. First, you'll need a wide-toothed comb to use on wet or damp hair. The widely spaced teeth allow you to comb through your wet hair, which is very vulnerable, without pulling, snagging, or breaking the hair.

The pocket comb is for men with short-to-medium hair to carry with them for styling throughout the day. (Men with long hair should always use only wide-toothed combs for the gentlest possible treatment of their hair.)

Combs should be made of plastic, hard rubber, or bone—never metal. When you run your thumb across the teeth of the comb, they should feel smooth to the touch. The ends should be rounded, never pointed—pointed ends can easily rip your hair and scratch your scalp.

Brushes

Men also need two types of brushes. The first is a vent brush, a plastic brush with rounded tips on very widely spaced bristles and an open back that looks like latticework. Because of the widely spaced bristles and the open back, more air flows into the hair, which gives you a fuller, fluffier look. A vent brush will also speed up your blow-dry time by allowing the air to move through the brush.

The rounded tips are very gentle and comfortable on the scalp.

The natural bristle combination brush is the other brush I recommend. Mason Pearson and Kent make good ones. This brush has two purposes. The first is to stimulate your scalp and loosen dead cells before shampooing. The second is to flatten and tame unruly hair. It can also be used during blow-drying to straighten wavy hair.

How to Dry Your Hair Naturally

Natural drying is best for eighty percent of all men. The trick to drying your hair naturally is to apply your body-builder or groomer, then shape your hair into place with either your fingers, a wide toothed comb, or a vent brush. Then don't touch your hair until it is dry, so it will dry into the right shape.

How to Blow-Dry Your Hair

What Type of Dryer to Use

The pistol-grip dryer is best. I don't recommend dryers that have brushes or combs attached, because the heat is too close to the hair and scalp and can easily burn or dry them out.

You really only need 1000 watts of power. More is not necessary. You should look for dryers that have a cool and warm setting, as well as hot. The warm setting is to dry your hair; the cool setting is to set your style and to close the cuticles of the hair, making it shinier.

Blowing Fullness into Your Hair

Fullness and lift result from the hair root standing vertically on the scalp. On damp hair that has been blotted with a towel to get most of the water

Don't spend more than five minutes with a blow dryer.

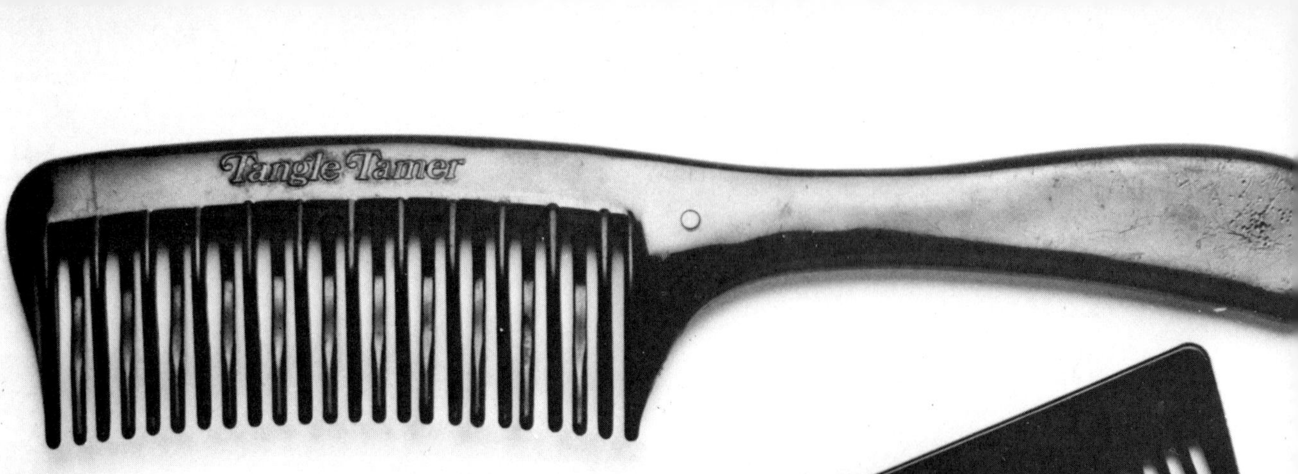

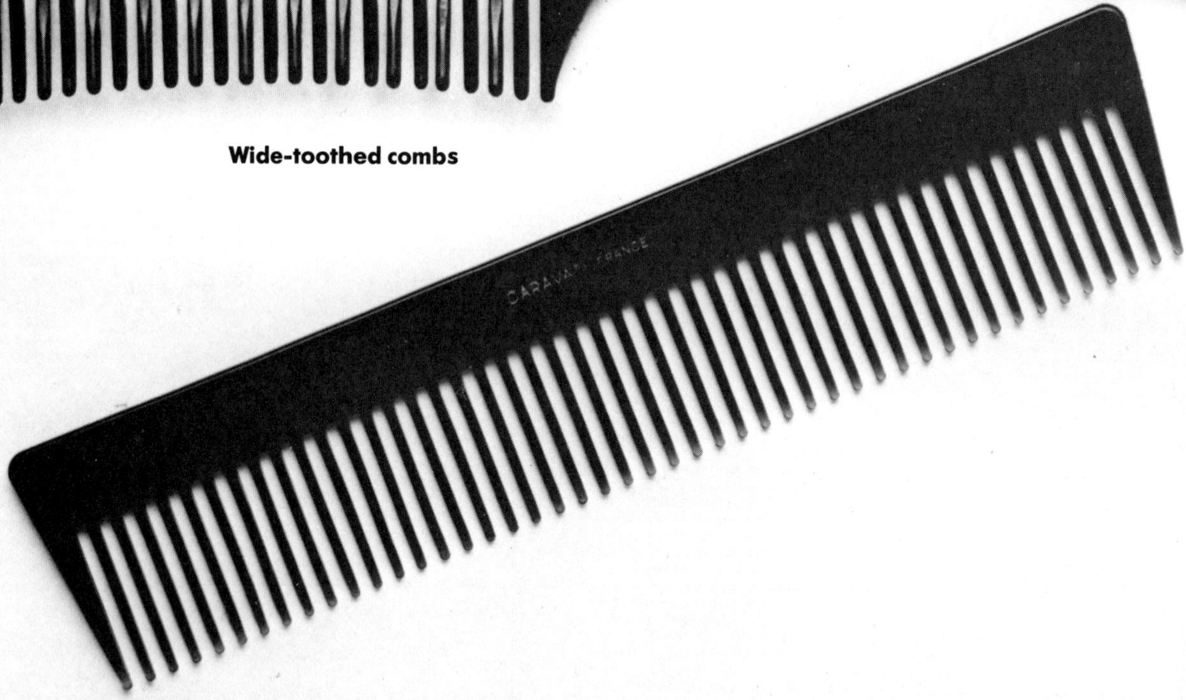

Wide-toothed combs

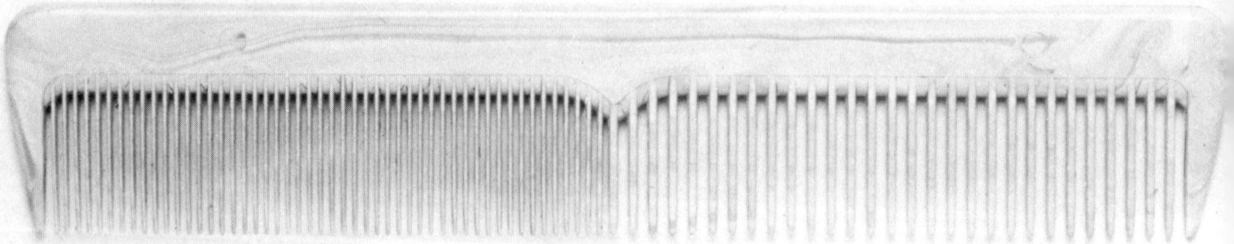

Fine-toothed combs

Combs and Brushes

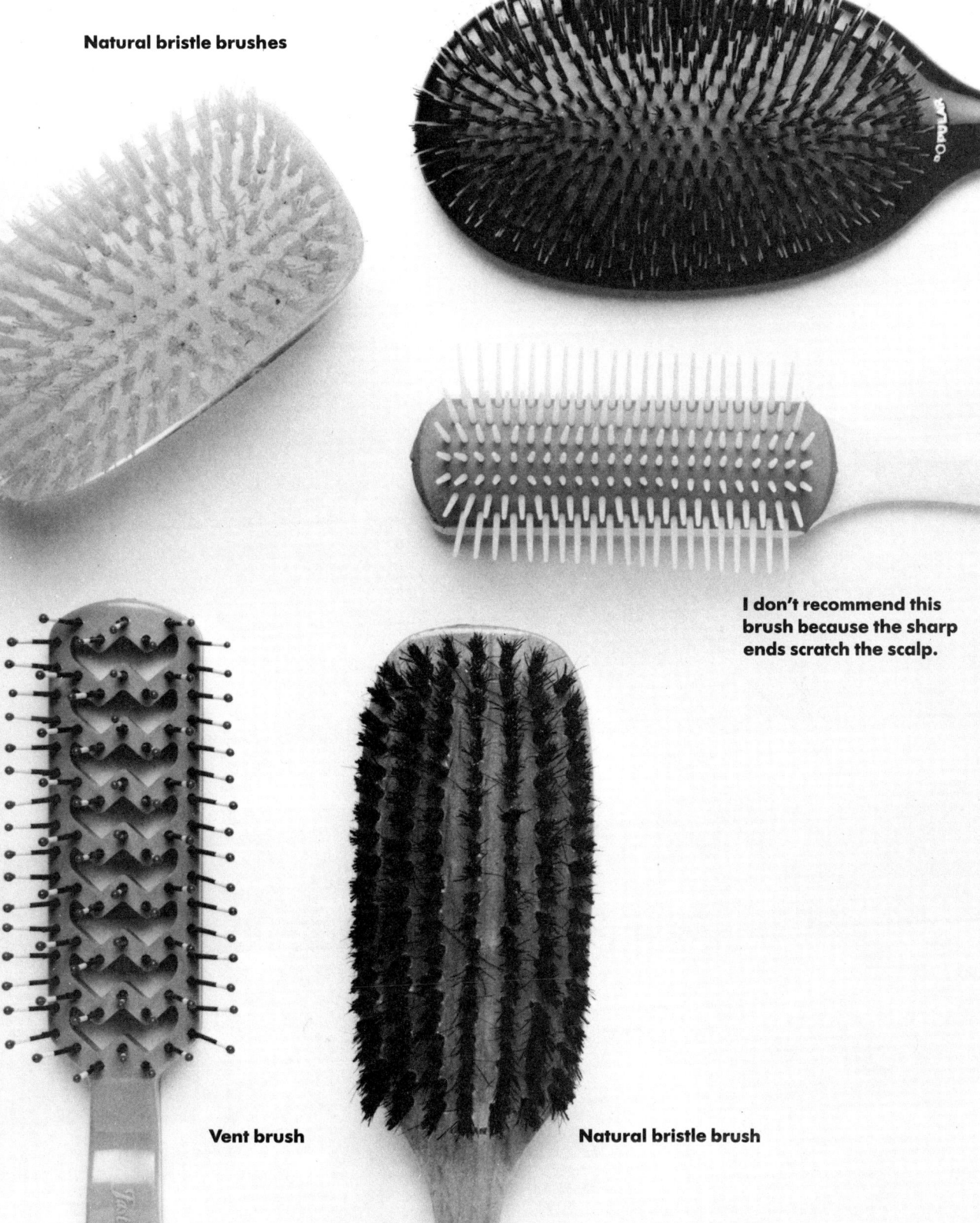

Natural bristle brushes

I don't recommend this brush because the sharp ends scratch the scalp.

Vent brush

Natural bristle brush

out, apply spray thickener setting lotion on the roots of the hair in the section where you want fullness. For instance, if you need fullness just on top, spray the roots of the hair on top of your head only.

Next, turn the dryer on to the warm or hot setting and, holding the dryer with one hand twelve to fourteen inches from the head, aim it at the roots of the hair. With the other hand, gently pull the hair upward. Do this all over the area where you want lift. This gets the hair to lift up off the head.

Now you need to give shape and direction to your style. With your vent brush, brush your hair into the direction you want it to go, and follow the brush with the cool air from your blow dryer. This will set the style and make your hair shinier. Cool air, like cool water, helps smooth the cuticle of the hair.

Blowing Wavy Hair Straight

Start with damp, towel-blotted hair, and put your dryer on the hot setting. Using a vent brush to direct the hair, blow all your hair forward toward your face until the hair is almost, but not totally dry.

Now take your combination brush and brush your hair straight back, following with the dryer on the warm setting. Turn the cold air on to brush your hair into the final shape. By brushing the hair forward, then back, you stretch out the wave in the hair. Then finish with cool air to lock in the new straight shape.

Blow-Drying Curly Hair

Curly hair looks best when dried naturally. But if you're in a hurry or the weather is cool and you

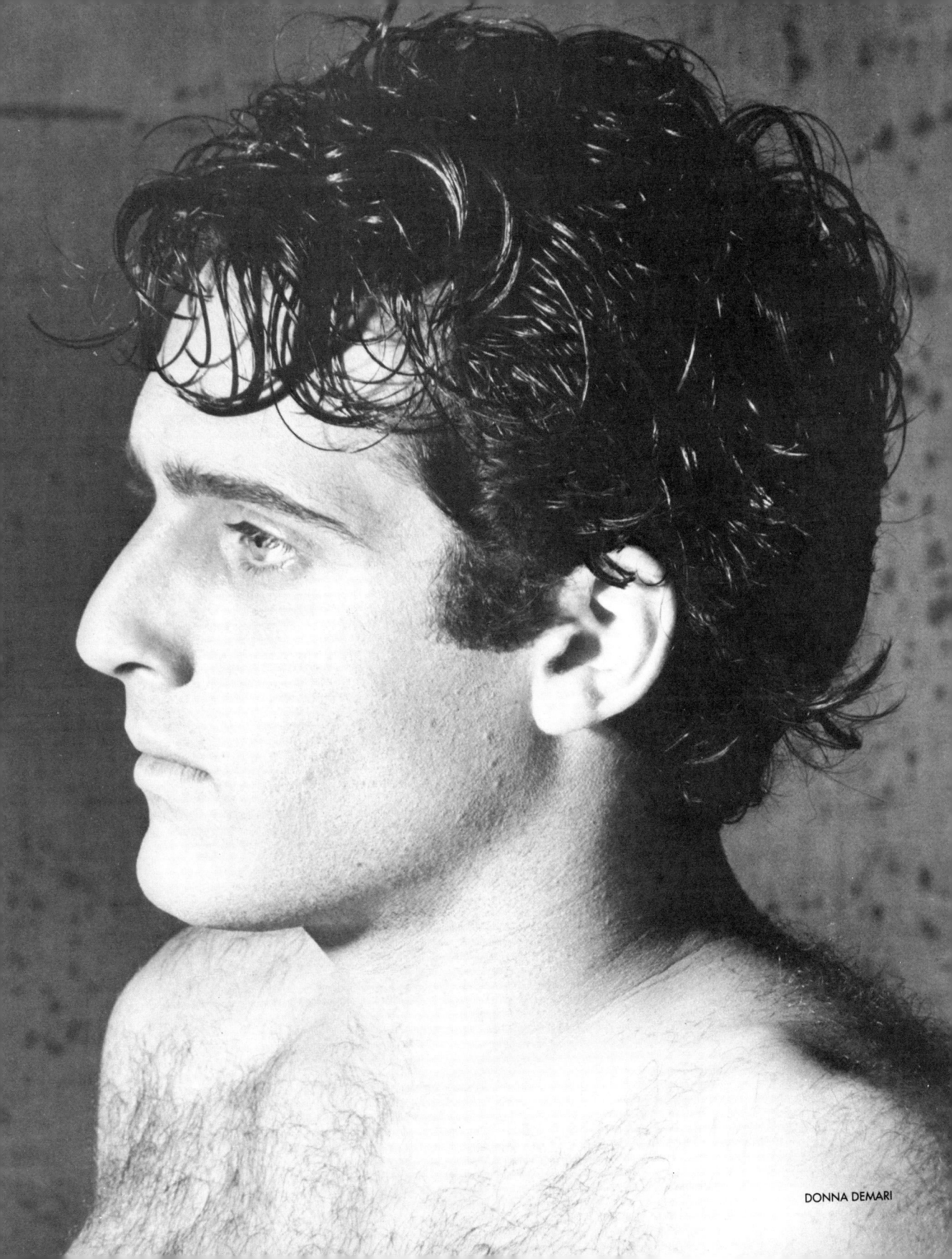

DONNA DEMARI

don't want to leave the house with wet hair, then you should use a blow dryer with a diffuser attachment.

The diffuser attachment looks like a shower head but larger; it attaches to the open end of your hair dryer. The air comes out through little holes rather then in a concentrated blast. This will dry your hair without blowing the curl out of it.

The key to no-fuss maintenance is a good basic cut. The shape of your hair should depend on this cut, not on your blow-drying technique or the groomer you put on your hair.

- If you have to depend on a grooming product, you have the wrong cut.
- If you spend more than fifteen minutes with a blow dryer, then you either have the wrong haircut or you are trying to make your hair go against its nature.

Use your hair's natural potential. It means more freedom and less maintenance time for you!

7.

THINNING HAIR AND HAIR LOSS

Use Proper Styling to Make the Most of What You Have

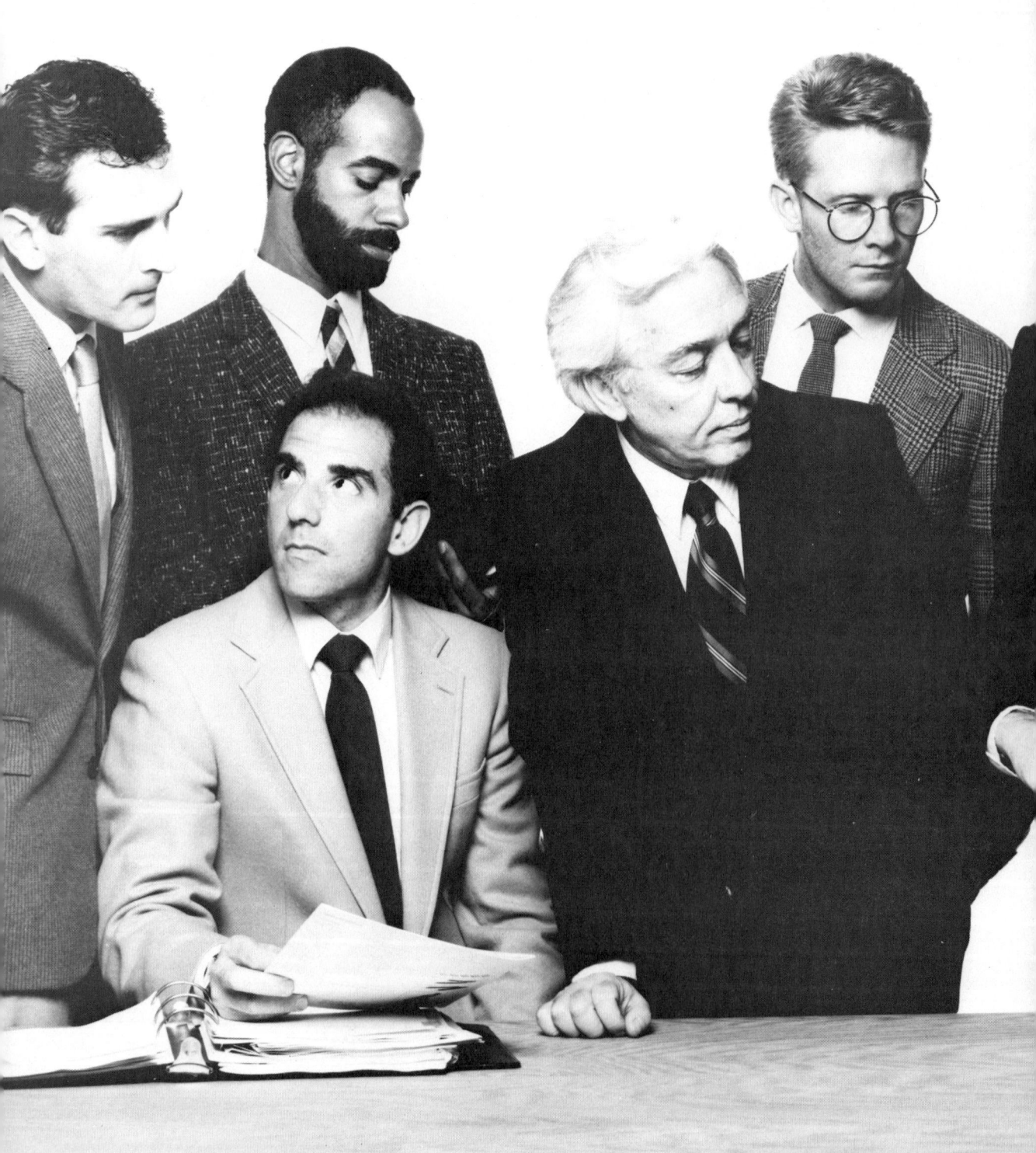

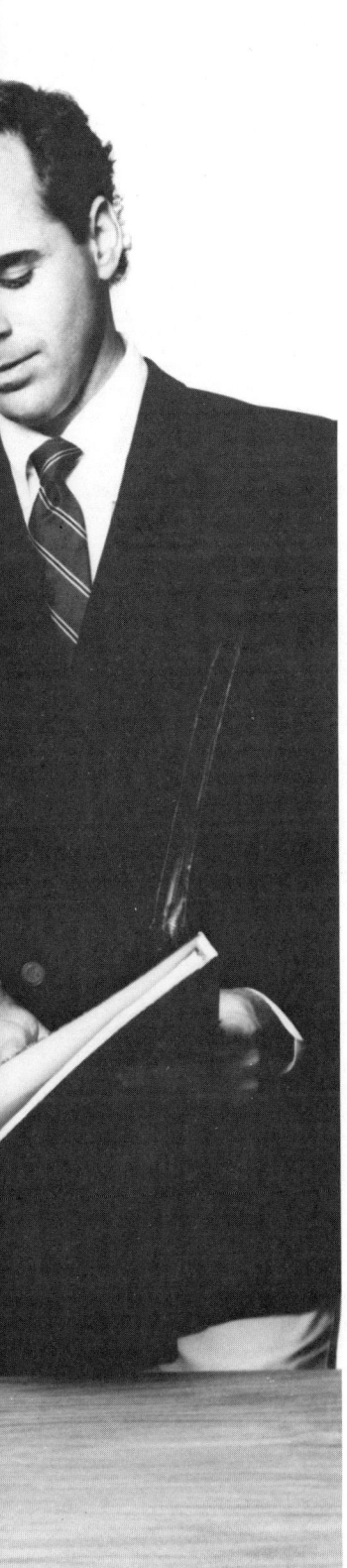

Room at the Top

No man wants to lose hair. We associate great-looking hair with some very important qualities—for example, sexuality, health, and youth. No wonder we care.

There are those who say that losing your hair is unimportant. Most men, including me, would disagree. But it's the way your hair *looks*, not how much of it you have, that really matters.

As I've said before, I like my job. I like making people feel better about themselves by making them feel good about their hair. As a hair stylist, I know that thinning hair can create havoc with your self-image. So I've tried over my entire career to find ways to make thinning hair look great. And I've done it. The techniques that follow work. Any man with thinning hair can get a good look, guaranteed. I'll show you how.

One basic secret: Don't panic. It is a fact that men lose their hair. Instead of counting the hairs in your drain, be happy with what you have. Hairs down the drain are gone forever, but you can make the hair that you have look better and thicker.

Do what you can. Make yourself look your best. Then leave your negative thoughts about thinning hair behind. Former President Gerald Ford, New York's Mayor Ed Koch, former Canadian Prime Minister Pierre Trudeau, and press lord Rupert

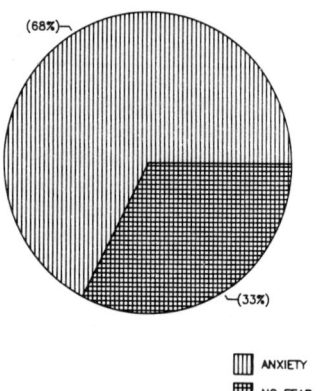

(68%)

(33%)

▯ ANXIETY
▦ NO FEAR

Murdoch are men of power and position who wear their baldness with confidence. So can you.

In the pages that follow, you will see all the ways to make thinning hair good-looking hair. There are many options. Just because your hair is departing, doesn't mean your self-image must follow. If you choose the right styling options, you might just look better than before. Truly!

Why Are You Losing Your Hair?

You lose your hair for the same reason that your nose is shaped the way it is and your feet are the size they are: genetic programming. And this same genetic programming may be why you do so well at your job, why you easily mastered tennis, or why women find your mouth so virile-looking, so don't feel that you've been cheated.

There are some circumstances under which hair loss might be caused by other than genetic coding—chemotherapy, high fevers, and thyroid malfunctions are possible culprits. So are such physical traumas as wearing a ponytail for years, burns, and overexposure to X rays. But most likely you simply have a much more common condition: male pattern baldness, or MPB.

Male Pattern Baldness

Why on earth would there be a pattern to the way a man goes bald? Nobody knows for sure, but the pattern is readily recognizable.

It starts at puberty, when a man's testes and adrenal glands begin manufacturing the male hormone, testosterone, which is responsible for most male sexual characteristics, including voice change, sex organ development, and sexual drive. It also determines hair distribution after puberty.

What happens is that after puberty an oversupply of testosterone triggers hair follicles to produce hair on some areas of the body while shutting down the production of other follicles. This is why a man can have a hairy *body* and a bald *head*. How this genetic programming works remains a mystery.

What is the "pattern" referred to in male pattern baldness? At puberty, the hair begins to recede in an M shape at the temple area. At the same time, but in varying degrees, a circular pattern of hair loss may begin at the crown of the head. The loss is slow in some cases, but too quick for comfort in others. The point of the M keeps receding. The bald spot at the crown widens. Eventually, the receding hairline joins the thinning crown, and all that remains is a horseshoe pattern of hair on the sides and back of the head. That's MPB. It's a natural part of manhood. It should be explained to young boys as they grow up, so it will come as no surprise or shock when it happens, and it can happen as early as sixteen or seventeen years of age.

Let's see how we can handle it.

What to Do about Thinning Hair

You can lose loads of hair before anyone notices and before the basic look of your hair changes dramatically. During the first years of MPB—perhaps for as much as eight or ten years—you can keep the look of your hair intact by making the hair you have look thicker. Here's how.

- **Shampoo frequently.**

If your hair is oily, it is heavy and lies down and sticks together. It looks thin. Frequent shampooing (every day if necessary) removes excess oil.

Thin hair can look fuller if handled properly.

Your hair shafts will stand away from the scalp and away from other hair shafts for a fuller look.

- **Use conditioners.**

Many hair conditioners coat hair shafts, giving each shaft some extra thickness. Both RK Shampoo and Conditioner (by Redken Laboratories) and Aramis Malt-Enriched Thickening Shampoo and Conditioner contain body-building proteins that give your hair the overcoating it needs.

These can work two ways. One is to coat the hair, like the plastic coating on your driver's license, with an invisible, body-building shield. Usually this is made of a special wax formula. Thicket, made by Madric, Ltd., is one of the best of this type. You just rub it through freshly shampooed, damp hair, then comb or brush the hair into place. Your hair will look slightly plastic when it dries, but a quick combing or brushing will fluff it up for a completely natural but much fuller look. Hair thickeners easily shampoo out of your hair. Don't expect them to give your hair all the benefits of a good conditioner. Their waxes don't provide the natural shine and manageability of protein-based conditioners.

I prefer another type of thickener, which has much better conditioning benefits. This contains animal proteins that are absorbed into the hair shafts in about five minutes, instead of simply lying on top of the hair strands. Thus the hair is "fattened" up naturally, with added shine and manageability. Mahdeen's MEDI-PRO, currently available only in beauty supply stores, is the best of this type. Follow the directions on the package.

- **Try moving your part.**

Stop and take a brand-new look at yourself.

After a shower, pat—don't rub—your hair dry. While your hair is damp, try wearing it with a different part. You get so used to seeing yourself with your hair parted on its usual side. Flip the part to the other side. Your hair will automatically have more lift because you're changing the root direction of the hair. Lift comes from the root of the hair. The results may surprise you. Just lowering or raising your part can make your receding hairline unnoticeable.

Please avoid the plastered down look! You've seen it and I've seen it, and it doesn't fool us or anyone else. A man with a balding top grows his side hair long, moves his part down close to his ear, and sweeps his long side hair up and over, plastering over his bald spot. Wet or windy days play havoc with this hairstyle . . . and your image.

Sometimes if you just tousle the hair and don't wear a definite part, your hair will look thicker. I encourage men to move their hair with their hands and not to comb and brush too much for styling. Move your hair with spread fingers. This will give the hair direction (left to right for example) and you'll get more lift. Anytime you comb or brush with too much pressure you flatten the hair. Your goal is to unflatten the hair.

Another way of wearing no part is simply to shake your hair when you get out of the shower and comb it with your fingers. You may notice that when your hair is left wild like this, it can camouflage your receding hairline.

- **Cut your hair shorter, overall.**

If you have a large, horseshoe-shaped bald spot on the top of your head, you have two options. You can cut your hair relatively close to the head, so it

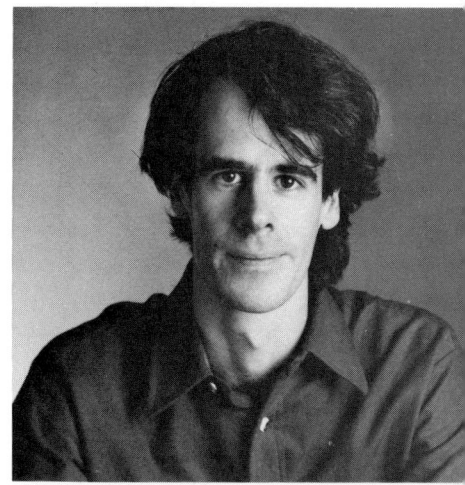

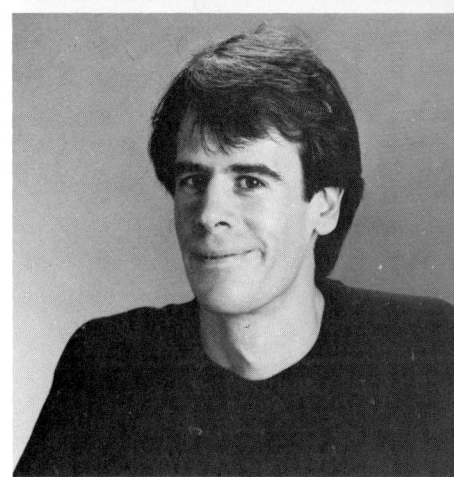

Long hair adds to the length of Taz's face. He had been cutting his own hair at home and knew he needed a wider shape. He needed a professional cut. Mid-length hair widens his narrow face. Ear exposure gives him cheekbones, and wispy bangs attract attention to his eyes. He blow-drys the back of his hair to keep his cowlicks from flipping out.

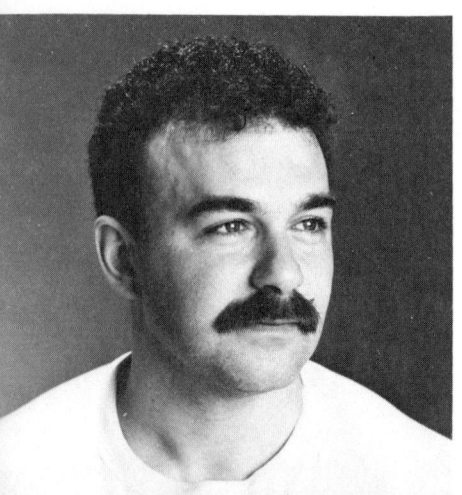

Tom makes his receding hair look thicker with a short haircut. Shorter hair adds bulk to any texture or amount of hair and shows off an athletic build. Tom's hair is very curly and dry. He uses an oily groomer to add shine and to help the cut keep its shape. His moustache draws attention away from his hairline to focus on the center of his face. Short hair at the sides of the head draws attention to his sparkling blue eyes.

is in proportion with your face (from half an inch to an inch). Your hair will then look neat and natural. You may then want to consider growing some facial hair to draw attention away from the top of your head to your face. Your other option is to replace the hair you have lost, which we will discuss later in this chapter.

- **Keep all your hair in proportion.**

Don't grow long hair on the back and sides of your head if the hair is thinning on top. It's much better to keep all your hair in proportion, because longer hair lies flat and limp under its own weight. The longer hair is, the more it weighs. Shorter hair always has more lift.

- **Use less creme rinse.**

Creme rinses can weigh the hair down. If you use only a dot, a dime-sized dollop, your hair will get the benefits of the creme rinse (shine, manageability) without the heaviness. Once a week, rinse your hair with a 50/50 mixture of lemon juice (or vinegar) and water. A quick one-minute rinse with this mixture will remove any heavy coating that might build up on the hair.

- **Change your hair groomer.**

If you're using one of the oily type groomers, such as Oily VO5, Brylcreem, or Clairol's Vitapoint, switch to a nonoily groomer (Dep, Tenax, Clinique's Hair Shaper, Aramis Multiplexx).

- **Try blow-drying with a setting lotion.**

This is the technique I invented for David Frost and mentioned in Chapter 1. You need a setting lotion, bristle brush, and blow dryer. When hair is damp, lift up half-inch sections and spray the setting lotion on the roots of the hair. Just spray the areas where you want more lift (usually the top). Use the blow dryer on medium heat. With one hand holding the dryer at least ten inches from your head, use the other hand to pull the hair upward lightly as you aim the air from the dryer at the roots.

Move from section to section quickly. Remember, you're working on the roots to get lift. After the root hair sections are dry, use a natural bristle or vent brush to push your hair in the direction you want it to go.

Like anything new, you have to practice. After a few times, you'll have this easy trick down pat.

- **Get a color rinse.**

You'll need a professional's help for this technique, but it may be well worth it. A solution of equal parts shampoo, twenty-volume peroxide, and hair color is applied to damp hair. It's left on about two to ten minutes, then rinsed out. Color rinses don't necessarily change the color of your hair—it depends on the shade of hair color used. They do, however, add body and lots of shine, which is just the right prescription for thinning hair.

- **Lighten your hair.**

A strong contrast between hair and skin tones can be dramatic, but for men with dark, thinning hair, the color difference between their hair and scalp is intense, magnifying the lack of hair density. Blonds and redheads can lose much more of their hair than a brunette can before it becomes noticeable.

By lightening your dark hair just a few discreet shades you can eliminate the strong contrast. Thinning hair becomes denser-looking.

- **Try some diversionary tactics.**

Any magician can tell you the secret of decep-

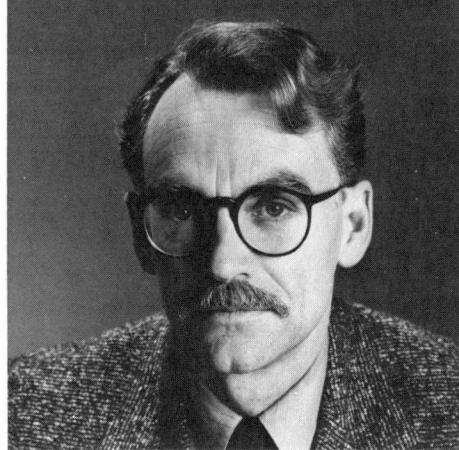

Don makes the most of his receding hairline. His hair is cut short at the sides to accentuate his eyes (even with glasses). The longer length on top plays up his natural wave. A well-trimmed moustache helps draw the eye away from the hairline and down toward the center of the face. To remove the yellowing buildup of shampoos and pollutants in the air and to keep his hair shiny, he rinses his hair after each shampoo with a mixture of lemon and water.

tion: Keep 'em looking the other way. Beards and moustaches do this. A flattering, sculpted bit of facial hair draws attention away from your head, focusing it down onto your face.

- **Get a body wave.**

A body wave is an easy way to give more fullness to the hair on top of your head. This wave will chemically alter your hair's structure, giving it more body and texture. Your hair stylist may wave only the hair on top of your head and then blend it more easily with the bulkier hair on the sides and back, or you could have a full body wave to make all the hair on your head thicker. The hair is then cut shorter on the sides and back to give it the look of overall equal proportions.

- **Stop worrying about your hair.**

So you're losing it. So what? Haven't you got a personality? A career? A good brain? A nice smile? It could be that you have been so preoccupied with your receding hair that you've been ignoring your good points.

Sean Connery goes on television shows all the time without his toupee. He's happy, healthy, and wears the hairpiece only in the movies. He's obviously not ashamed to go in public *au naturel.*

My first advice to you if you are losing your hair is to *start shaping up the rest of you.* If a well-dressed man with a beautifully fit body comes into a room, looking happy and healthy, the last thing anybody is going to notice about him is whether he has a bald spot.

Hair Again

If you have tried the techniques mentioned above and your thinning hair or baldness is still

Being bald can mean confidence. Just look at his eyes.

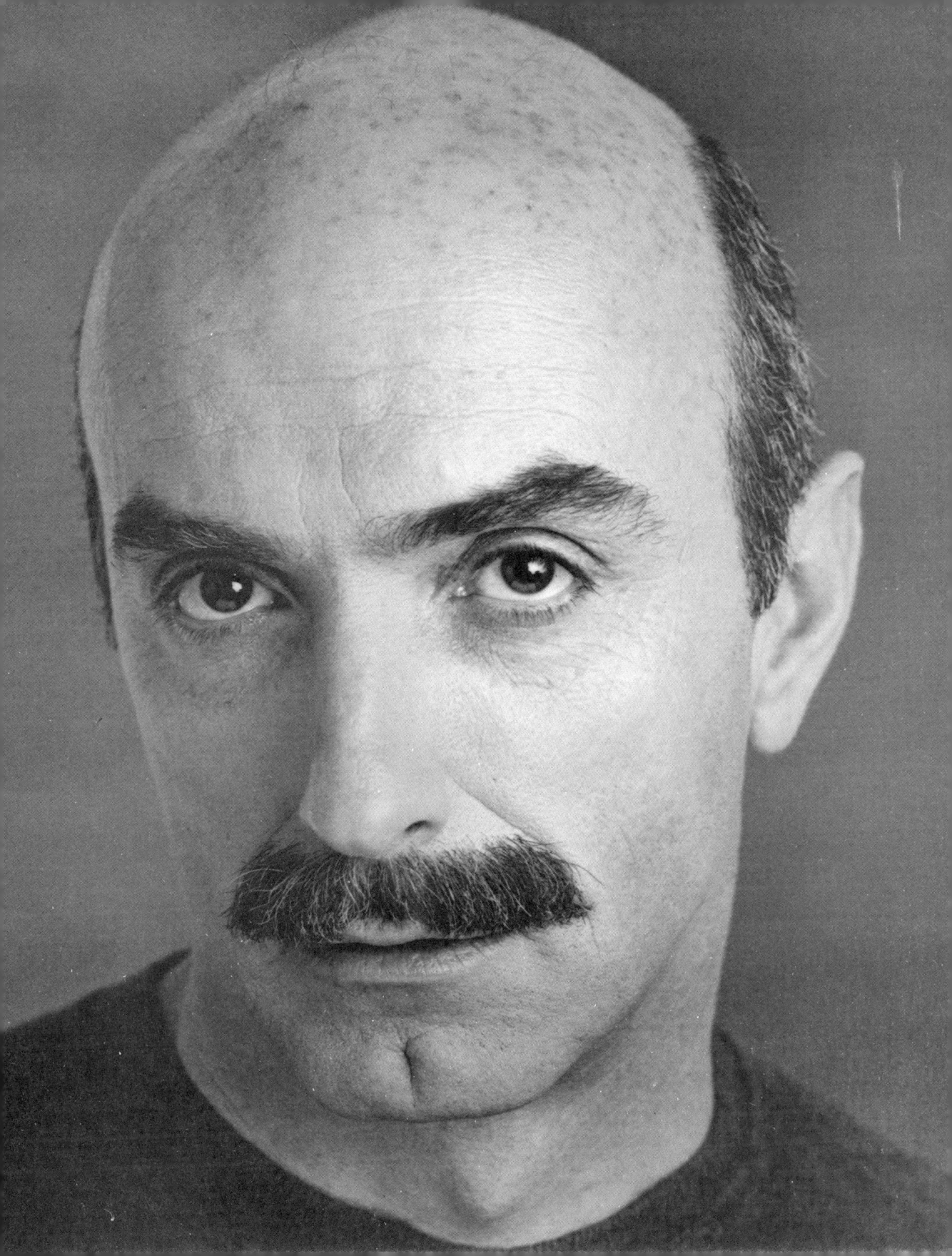

making you miserable, then there is no reason not to replace the hair you've lost. That's what handling your hair is all about.

What follows is the latest information on hair replacement, from hairpieces to transplants. The pros and cons of each are considered. Correctly chosen and used, hair replacements will give you back what nature has taken away. If this kind of help would please you, then go for it.

All about Hairpieces

The Good News

Ricardo Montalban, William Shatner, and Burt Reynolds (in most of his movies) all wear hairpieces. And they all—the hairpieces and the men—look great.

A hairpiece gives the illusion that you have an enviable head of hair. But *all* the components must be right: design, fit, cut, and color. When they are properly matched, your hairpiece will look very good. But when they aren't, your hairpiece won't work in your behalf.

Avoid these pitfalls:

- *Too much hair.* Any man past his mid-twenties who has a head of hair that's too full attracts undue attention. The look is even more artificial on middle-aged men.

- *Too dark in color.* Your skin and hair lose some of their pigment as you age. If your hair is too dark in relation to your skin tone, your hairpiece will look artificial.

- *Too low a hairline.* Some receding of the hairline is common to all men as they age.

If you are going to wear a hairpiece, then buy yourself the best. Forget stretch wigs or anything you can order through the mail.

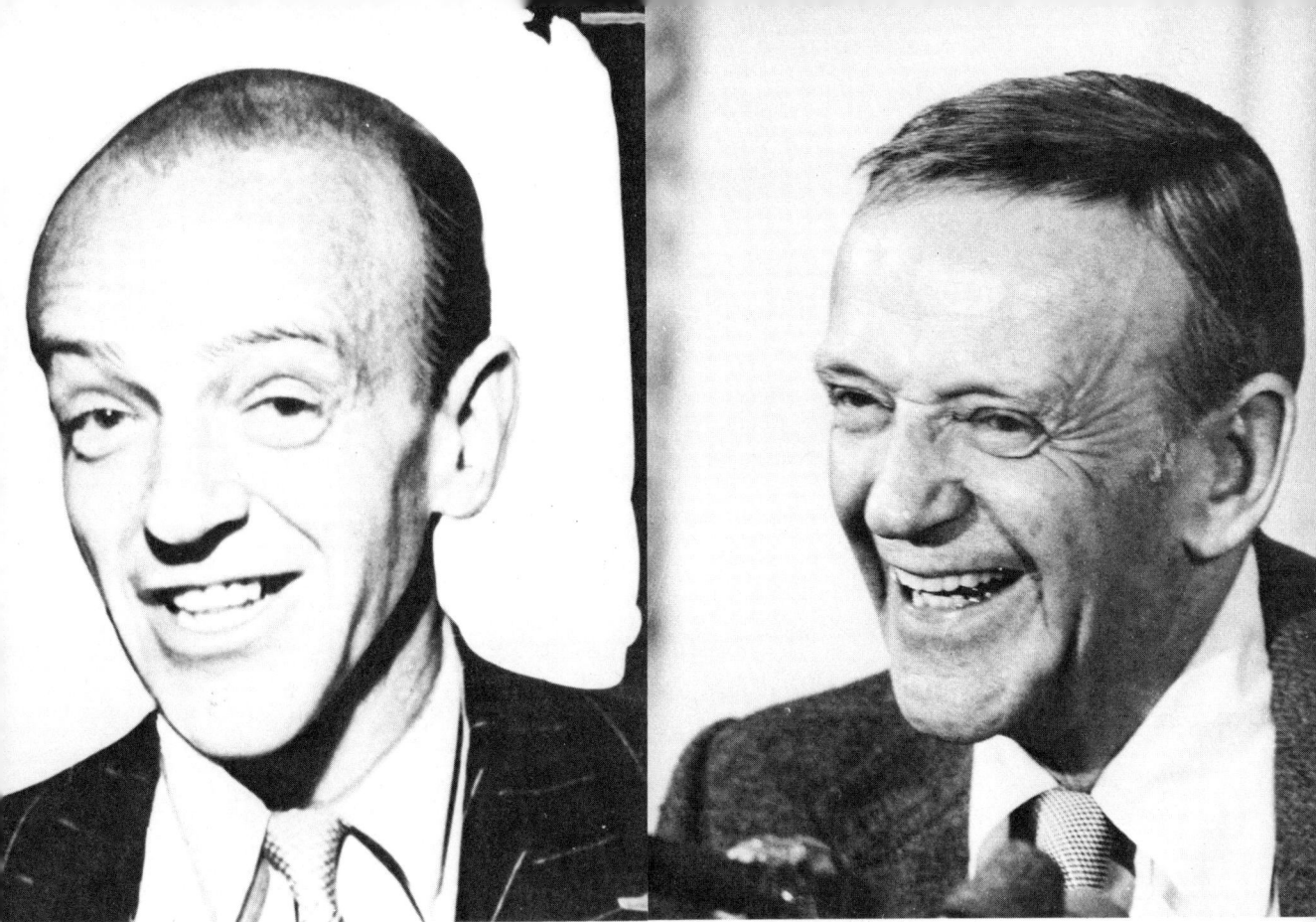

The King of Style knows his look.

Fred Astaire's lean line was well thought-out, from his dancing feet up! His hair was always thin and fine. Besides giving the look of the times, keeping his hair short also worked best for his dancing image, offering no distraction from his total silhouette. His hairpiece carries on the uncluttered dancer's line—not too thick, with a believable color and hairline. It's realistic and perfect for Fred.

159

Shop around for a barber or hair stylist who specializes in hairpieces. He or she will measure your bald area—its contours, size, and shape. He or she will then cut some samples of your own hair to color match with the human or synthetic hair being used for the piece. That will then be sewn onto a base.

Your final hairpiece should fulfill the following criteria:

- It should contain mostly human hair. This type of hairpiece is far more expensive than one composed all of synthetic fibers but well worth it. The natural texture and color of human hair has never been duplicated. So I recommend no more than twenty percent synthetic hair in a hairpiece, if any at all.

- It should have many different shades of color, just like your natural head of hair. To match your own hair, at least three or four different shades should be used.

- The base of the hairpiece should be made of a lightweight ventilated material that looks somewhat like lace. This kind of base is healthiest and most comfortable because it allows air to reach your scalp. The base should be molded to conform to the contours of your head.

- For the most foolproof appearance, the right hairline construction is vital. The best hairpieces have hairlines of very fine, almost transparent lace, with the hairs carefully placed for the most natural effect. The dead giveaway of a badly made hairpiece is a hairline with too much hair, uniformly placed.

- Hair should be sewn by hand to the base.

With hand sewing, individual hairs can be spaced properly, creating a more natural appearance.

A fine quality hairpiece may cost about $1,000 and take about two weeks to construct. You wouldn't want a contractor to skimp on time in building an addition to your home, so you should be suspicious of anyone who will make you a hairpiece in less than a week. When your new hair is ready, you will secure it to your head using double-faced surgical tape. You will have your hair back . . . and you may just walk a little taller.

The Bad News

Most of the negatives associated with hairpieces can be summed up in a word: inconvenience. First of all, you can't just put on a hairpiece as if it were a favorite old sweater and weat it day in and day out. The piece should be removed nightly and your scalp washed to keep it bacteria-free. Also, you're going to have to buy two hairpieces, because one will periodically be "in the shop" every few weeks for cleaning, styling, or needed repairs.

Activities such as swimming are at best risky. Submerging your hair in public could end in embarrassment.

Even good quality hairpieces (the only kind you should consider) last only about as long as a couple of sets of tires. It is doubtful that even the best, most carefully maintained piece will see a fifth birthday.

Make the most of what you have *before* taking drastic measures.

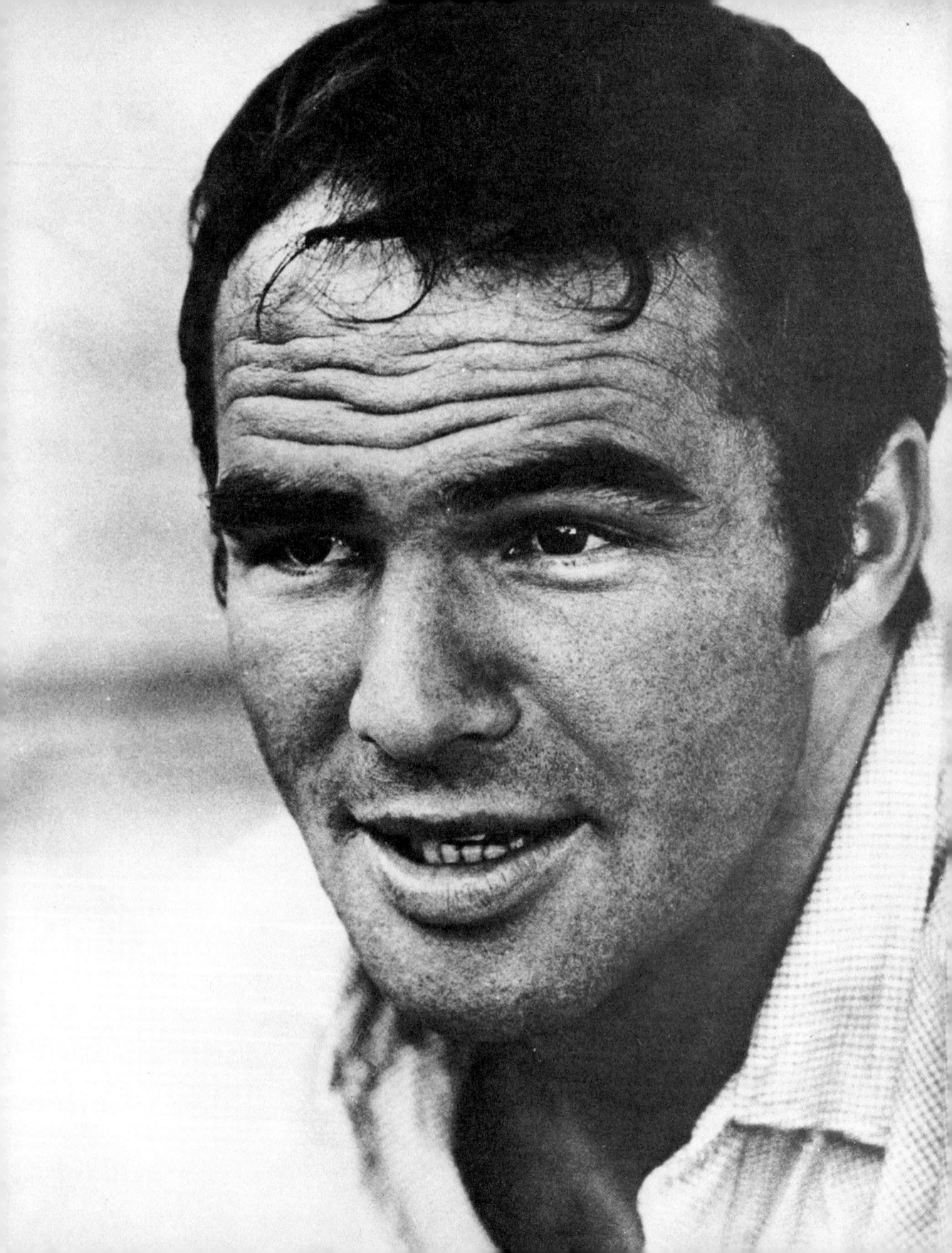

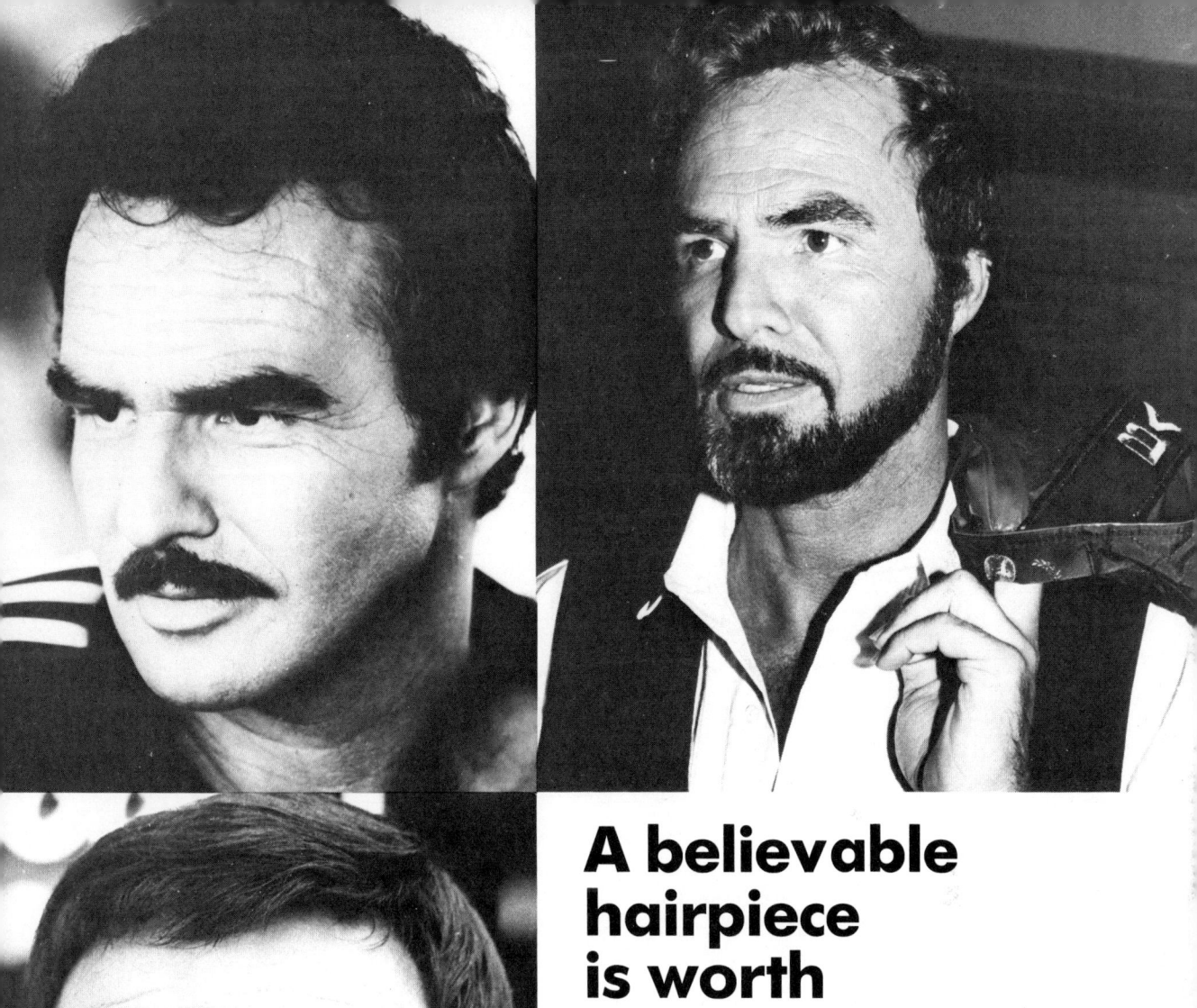

A believable hairpiece is worth the expense.

In the early photo, male pattern baldness is happening to Burt Reynolds. A well-made hairpiece brings back the full head of hair, which adds to his sexy image. Notice the soft line of the front hairline—essential in a good hairpiece. The moustache balances his intense eyes.

AP/WIDE WORLD PHOTOS

Get several opinions before electing surgery.

Drastic Measures

Hairweaving and suture implants are methods that try to make hairpieces permanent, so that you can treat them more like natural hair. This is a great idea, but both methods fall short in execution.

Hairweaving is by far the least harmful. In order to anchor a hairpiece to the head, a semicircular braid is made from the horseshoe-shaped fringe hair on the sides and back of your head. The hairpiece is then tied to this braid. The problem with this method is that tight braiding can cause fringe hair to loosen and fall out. Also, because the scalp is covered for weeks at a time, it can't be cleaned nearly as thoroughly as the daily washing a taped hairpiece allows.

While hairweaving is just a bad idea, suture implants are absolutely horrific. Often advertised by "clinics" using medical-sounding terminology (a "miraculous surgical process," etc.), implants are stitches or sutures sewn into the scalp and tied into rings to form, like woven hair in hairweaving, "anchors" for attaching a hairpiece.

Under certain circumstances, sutures can be ripped out of the scalp, causing not only embarrassment, but a great deal of bleeding and pain. In addition, the risk of bacterial infection is very real, as surgical sutures were never intended to remain in the skin. Finally, such sutures leave scars. If you ever decide to go natural again, you will have to make up a very good story to cover your tracks.

Hair Transplants

Though I cannot, in all good conscience, recommend hair transplants, sutures, or anything that involves surgery on the scalp, close to a million and a half people have undergone successful hair transplants since the mid-1950s.

The punch graft method is the most common transplant procedure. You go to the doctor, usually a dermatologist, after growing your hair long enough to cover your transplant sites. You'll have shampooed that morning (you won't be able to shampoo again for two days). You'll have eaten a very light breakfast and planned to stay home after the procedure.

On the first of three sessions, a one-by-three-inch rectangular area is trimmed from the back of your head, where you still have a good growth of hair. From this section, forty donor grafts will be removed and transplanted to wherever hair is needed.

A local anesthetic will be injected into the donor and bald areas. The doctor will use a punch that looks like a cookie cutter attached to a high speed drill. He'll then extract the grafts from the host area and plant them in your balding areas. This takes about forty-five minutes.

Each of the donor grafts contains about eight to fifteen hairs. Ninety to ninety-five percent of them can be expected to grow. After the grafts are in place, a pressure dressing is applied. This will be removed when you return to the doctor's office the next day.

Within a month, the transplanted hairs will fall out, but within three months, permanent hair growth will begin. After two more transplant sessions your bald spot should be somewhat filled in. But be aware that:

- You will not have a thick head of hair. A thin

AP/WIDE WORLD PHO

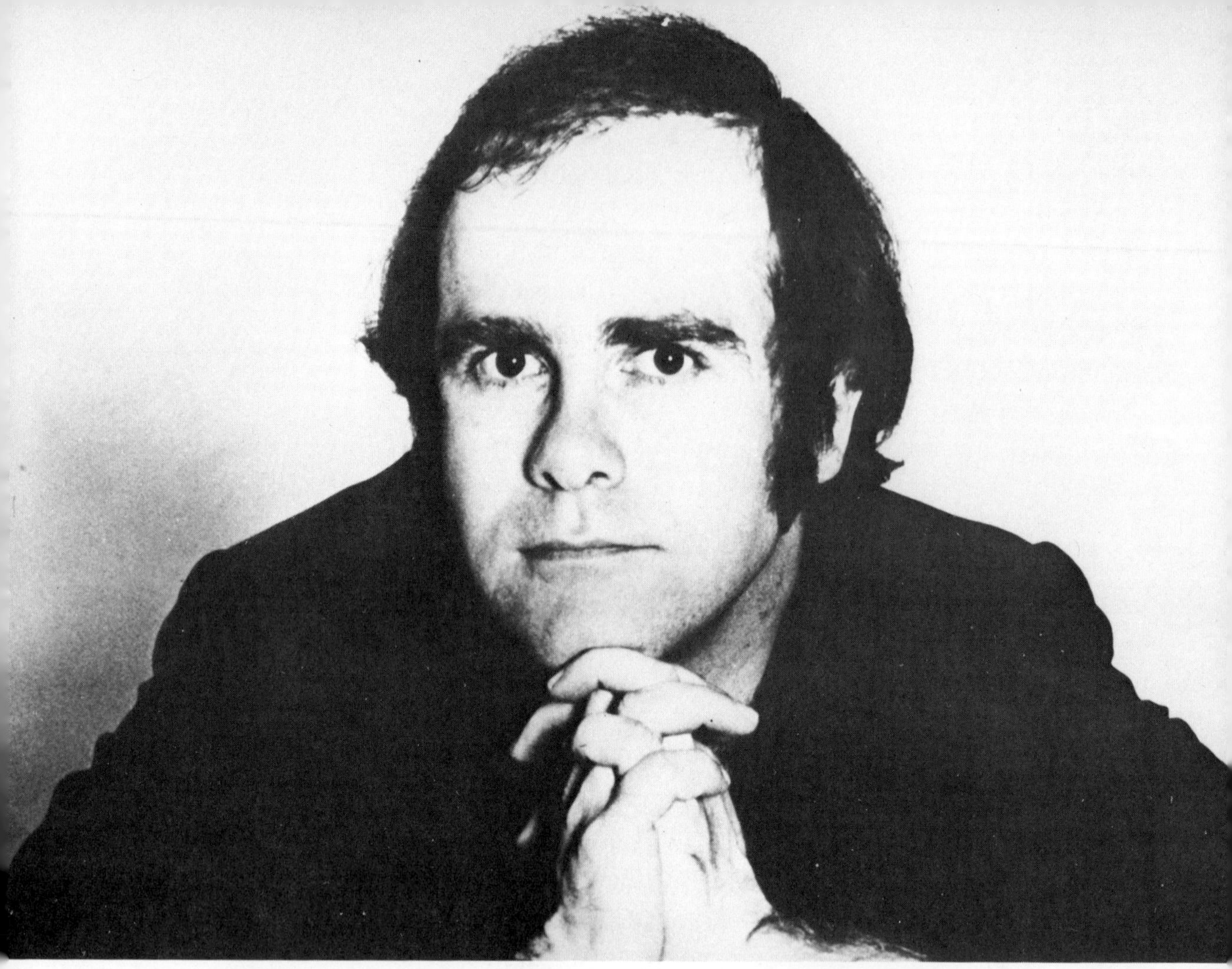

Transplants: Some have tried them.

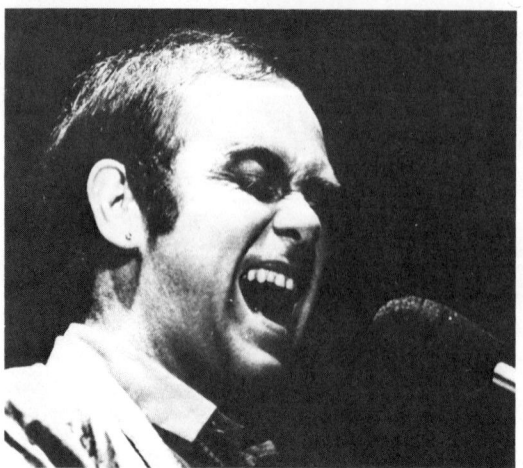

Elton John is among the tens of thousands of men who have undergone hair transplant surgery in the United States. It is classified as major surgery, and results may not be as fulfilling as you planned. Most men who have transplants eventually cut their hair short. Transplants will never restore your full hairline.

covering is all you can expect. You can, however, replace a receding hairline, which can make you look years younger.

• Your hair still might not look natural. Since the grafts can't be placed too close together (or they might not have a good blood supply), your hair might have the look of a newly planted lawn.

• Transplant sessions must be scheduled about two months apart, so it may take a year or more to complete the entire procedure. During this time your appearance will be marred by scabs and possible bleeding of the scalp.

• Not everyone has enough or the right kind of fringe hair to furnish the donor grafts. The hair must be relatively dense and coarse to give good coverage. Light hair is better than dark-colored locks.

• The cost may be prohibitive. The punch graft procedure cost is based on the cost per plug, ranging from $40 to $50. It may take up to five hundred plugs to get the results you're after. (If you're lucky, it can take as few as one hundred.) Figure between $4,000 and $11,000 for the whole procedure, a heady price for a head of hair. It can be tax deductible, but very few insurance plans will cover transplant operations.

Scalp Flaps

Another technique to create a new hairline uses a flap of hairbearing scalp, which is then moved to cover a bald area. It is sutured in place and soon begins to grow a new hairline.

With this procedure, the surgeon can transfer a larger amount of hair than with punch grafts—one scalp flap usually equals 350 punch grafts. Since the hair in the flap doesn't undergo the same trauma as the hair in punch grafts, there is almost immediate coverage and no shedding of hair before regrowth begins. The regrowth should be uniform in color, density, and texture over the entire head. (Sometimes punch grafts create differences in these characteristics in the implant area.)

On the other hand, the scalp flap operation is a delicate, more technically demanding procedure than punch grafts. The patient usually remains in the hospital for a week. Two such operations are usually needed, and the surgeon may charge from $2,000 to $5,000, excluding hospital expenses.

Scalp Reduction

Here's another risky procedure. It involves stretching the scalp over your bald spot. A surgeon cuts a rectangular strip of bald skin from the top of the scalp. He then stretches the hairy scalp over this opening and sutures it into place. This may not entirely cover the bald area, but it will greatly reduce it, and the remaining bald area can be filled in with implanted plugs of hair.

Scalp reductions are most often used when donor hair is limited, but the scalp must be loose enough to be stretched. The operation can be done under local anesthesia in the doctor's office and you can return to work within a day. The procedure takes about sixty minutes; it costs about $1,600 . . . or more.

Bear in mind that this operation requires a surgeon with great skill, or you risk such problems as raised scars, an unnatural direction of hair growth, or a relaxation of the scalp, which can leave a man's head nearly as bald as before his surgery.

Go for Quality

If you insist on surgical procedures, you *must* choose your surgeon with great care. *Never* go to a hair replacement "clinic" that offers you lower prices. These are often operated by nonmedical businessmen who hire physicians to perform the procedures. The clinic owner then takes a percentage (usually twenty percent) of the surgical fee.

I suggest making consultation appointments with three or four doctors who are experienced in hair replacement surgery. A plastic surgeon or a dermatologist who is a member of the American Society of Dermatologic Surgery is your best bet. (The society will provide you with a list of its members. Write to 210 South Grand Avenue, Suite 307, Glendora, California 91740.)

Ask your prospective doctors to let you talk with former clients. Looking at "before" and "after" hair transplant photographs is not a sure enough way to make a decision on something as important as surgery.

A Hair-Raising Pill?

Is there any vitamin, hormone, or drug that will outfox your MPB genes? We keep hoping for a medical miracle. Meanwhile, I find lotions, potions, and pills highly suspect.

As we went to press with this book, the most highly publicized new treatment for baldness involved a drug called Minoxidil, originally formulated to combat hypertension. Manufactured by the Upjohn Company, Minoxidil was found to produce new hair growth when taken orally. The "Catch 22" is that the new hair grows all over the body. Researchers are now experimenting with a

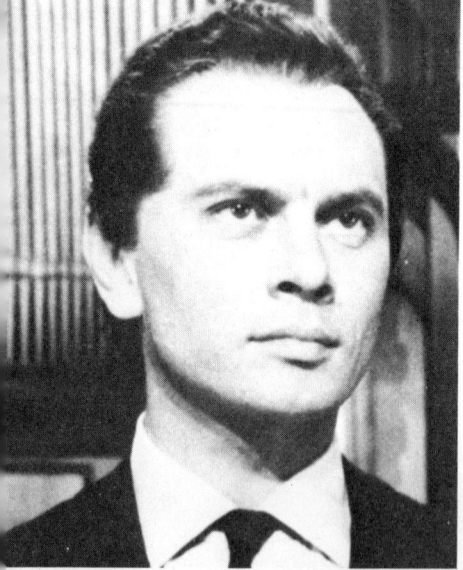

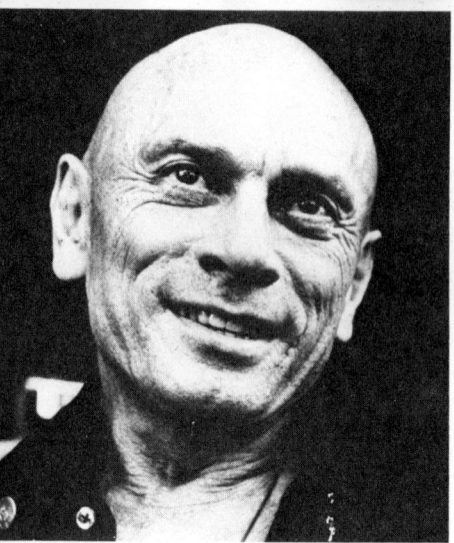

Yul Brynner shaved a full head of hair to play the leading role in The King and I. *The totally bald look is traumatic for many men but not for Yul. His confident masculinity was all the more apparent. He has continued to shave his head for over twenty years.*

Minoxidil ointment that is rubbed directly on the scalp, presumably to avoid the "hairy elbow" syndrome.

But what about all those therapies you have read about or for which you have seen advertisements? Vitamins for the hair? Hormones applied to the scalp? Scalp massagers?

Recently, a panel of medical scientists met in a special advisory panel to the United States Food and Drug Administration to review all the over-the-counter products that claim to prevent hair loss or to grow new hair. The products were intensively analyzed to find out which were safe and which worked. Many were safe (i.e., harmless). Not one worked.

Save your time. Save your money. Save yourself a load of frustration. Ignore the ads and the come-ons promising to prevent hair loss or to promote new growth. Set yourself free to concentrate on what *will* work for you.

Final Thoughts on Thinning Hair and Baldness

To repeat, here are the keys to living with male pattern baldness: Realize that MPB is a natural result of your manhood, use products that make your hair look thicker, get the right hair cut, and most importantly, *relax*. If you can't feel comfortable without your former hair, do something about the situation, but make sure *you* keep control of your looks.

8

FACIAL HAIR AND SHAVING

A Great, Close Shave Is Simply a Matter of Technique

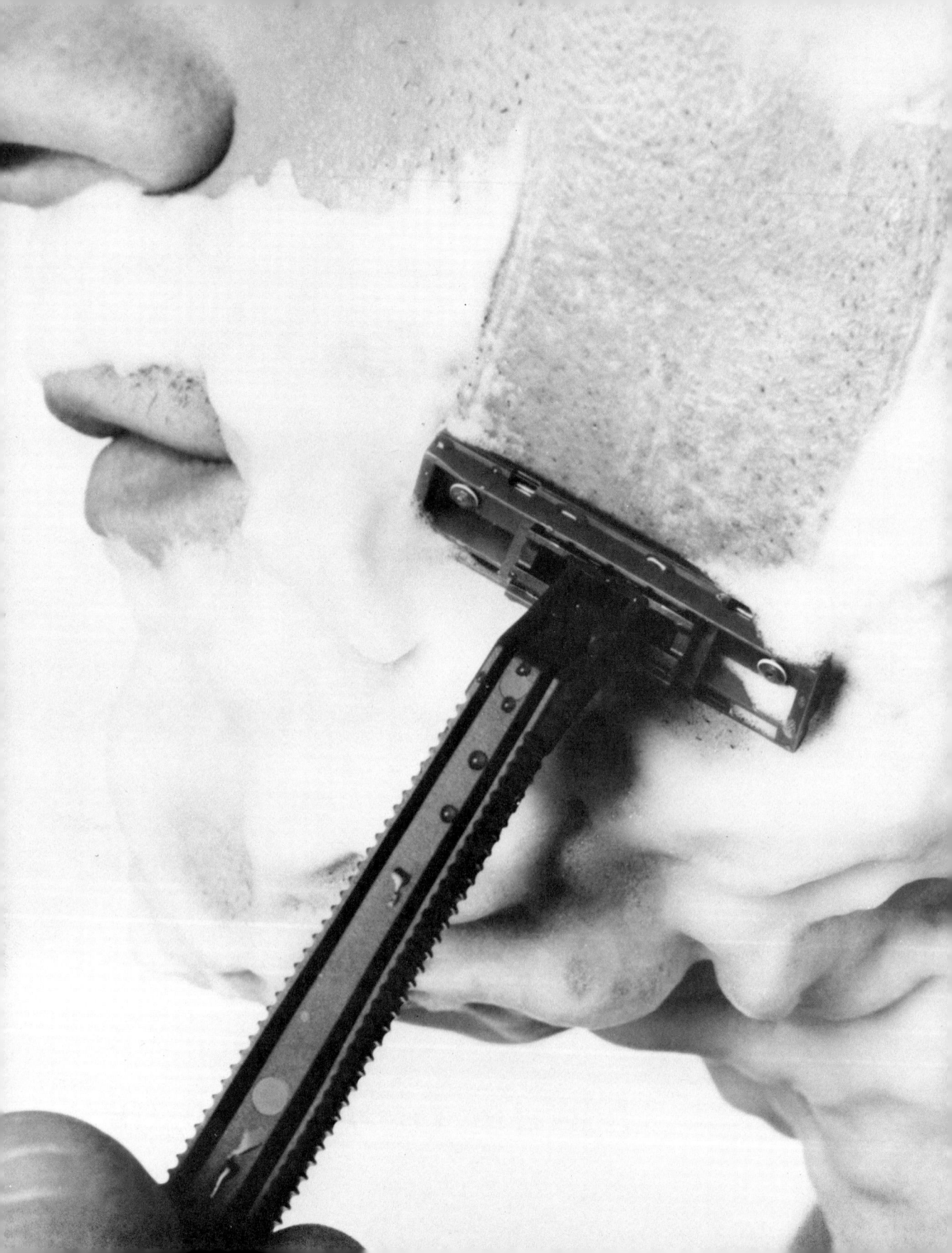

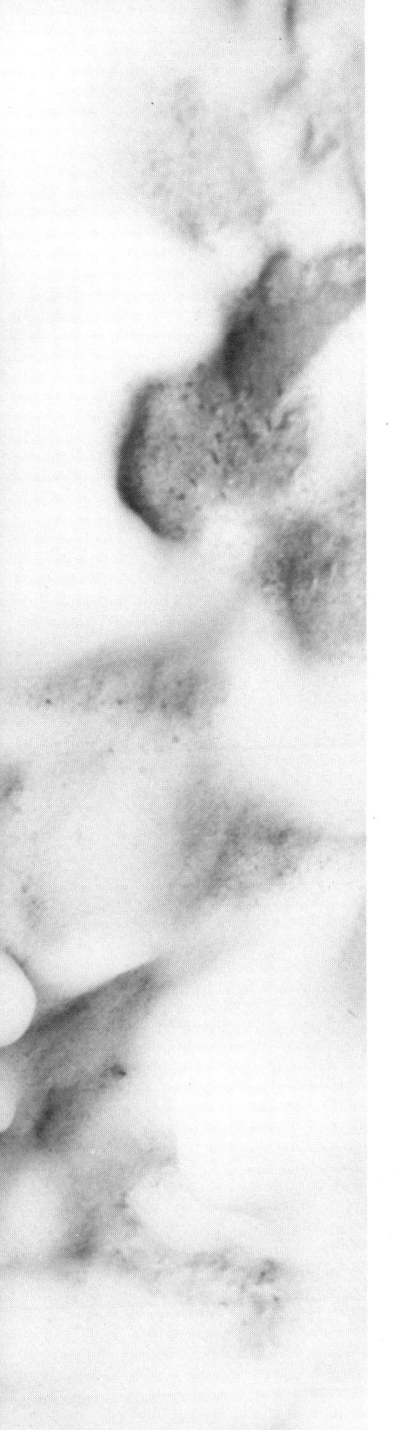

Face It: Shaving Takes Time

A man's facial hair is about as strong as copper wire of the same thickness, yet most men treat shaving as a chore requiring no more thought than taking out the garbage. So it's no surprise that problems such as nicks, cuts, and razor burns develop.

There is really no need for any of the problems associated with shaving. Today there are enough good products out there to give any man a great shave. But such a shave is more than just a matter of getting the whiskers off your face. Shaving should be an extremely important, integral part of your grooming routine.

The whole trick is not to rush. Shaving should be done in steps. Going through the extra effort to get a great shave may take three or four more minutes of your day, but you'll be thoroughly pleased by the results.

The Blade vs. the Electric Shaver

Advertising by the manufacturers of electric razors notwithstanding, shaving with a blade is the best way to remove your whiskers. Shaving with a blade delivers the three qualities most associated with quality beard removal; it's clean, close, and comfortable.

One problem associated with electric razors is their tendency to create ragged ends on facial hair shafts. Electric razors work by shearing whiskers—facial hair enters the perforated metal head or heads of the razor, where it's cut by moving blades positioned inside. Shaving experts say this can produce more ingrown hairs, because facial hair shafts are left sharper. If they happen to curve back toward the face they can cause irritation. You have less chance of developing ingrown hairs if you use a blade. I'll go into more detail about ingrown hairs later.

However, electric razors certainly have a place. Keep one in the file cabinet at work for unexpected dinner engagements. Use one when you travel or on those mornings when you are really in a hurry. But for your regular morning shave, you should use a blade for the best shave possible.

Most opinions show that the wet shave is a closer shave. If you have a very heavy beard (as does Richard Nixon who reportedly shaves at least two times daily), you might opt for a wet shave in the morning and a dry shave in the evening. Although wet shaving also helps to remove dead skin cells from the surface, too much shaving will cause irritation and rashes.

Getting the Best from a Blade Shave

There's no magic to getting a clean, close, comfortable shave with a blade. So why do so many men have problems? Most problems stem from approaching shaving as a task to be rushed through.

The First Step: Presoftening

Softening your beard is crucial to your shave, and there is only one way to do it right: with plenty of hot water. Dry facial hair is steely. Wet whiskers

The Five Steps:

1. **Softening your beard**
2. **Moisturizing**
3. **Applying a preshave product that helps further soften the beard and lubricate the skin so your razor will glide while cutting**
4. **Cutting the whiskers with the right razor in the right manner**
5. **Following your shave with the right after-shave skin protection routine**

are much more pliant because, when soaked, whiskers absorb water; they become swollen and weaker. Hot water promotes the softening action, in turn decreasing the resistance to the blade's cutting action.

You should splash on hot water for two minutes before applying anything else. Better yet, take a hot shower before shaving. Wash your face to clean your beard and remove facial oils.

Step Two: Moisturizing

I advise using a moisturizer before using a pre-shave product. This is an extra step that gives your skin extra protection. You can use any unscented body lotion—scented lotions contain alcohol, which dries the skin—or a moisturizer like Clinique's M lotion.

Step Three: Using the Right Preshave Product for Your Beard

After your whiskers have been softened with water, your next step in attaining the ultimate shave is to apply the right preshave product to your beard. A whole range of these products awaits—shaving soaps, shaving creams, brushless creams, and aerosol foams and gels.

Preshave products lubricate your skin so your razor will glide across your face. They'll lock moisture into your whiskers, keeping them soft and ready for shaving, and they'll help hold whiskers upright, plumping them up ready for the razor.

Each preshave product has unique benefits. Aerosol shave creams are by far the most popular, but another type might be better for you. Here are the pros and cons of each.

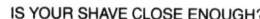

IS YOUR SHAVE CLOSE ENOUGH?

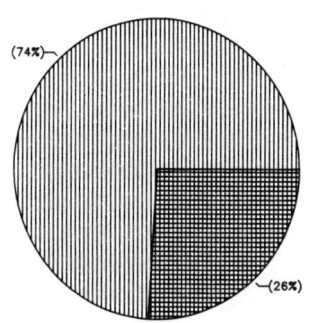

(74%)

(26%)

YES

NO

Shaving Soaps. You may think these are a throwback to Granddad's days, but they have merit today, too. Shaving soaps are basically bath soap with other ingredients added to help lubricate the skin and keep it from drying out. Such soaps also help prevent water from evaporating from your facial hair during shaving.

I recommend shaving soap for all but *dry skin*. (Any type of soap is drying to a degree, and you want to keep your skin as moist as possible.)

Good shaving soaps are Old Spice Shaving Mug Soap and Colgate Cup Soap. You'll need a shaving brush to lather them up. Look for a badger hair brush. It costs more, but it works best and lasts for years.

Lathering shave creams. Lathering shave creams are basically soft shaving soaps that come in a tube. You squeeze the soap onto your fingers, apply it to your face, and use a shaving brush or your fingers to lather up your cheeks, chin, and neck. A good one is Noxzema Medicated Shave Cream.

Brushless shave creams. This is the most widely used type of nonfoam preshave. It has recently become more popular. Several makers of quality men's toiletries have offered it as an alternative to foamy shaving creams.

You apply brushless shaving creams directly to your wet face from the tube. Rather than foaming, the cream simply coats the face with rich emollients and moisturizers. This provides extremely good lubrication for your skin, so that your razor really glides, reducing the risk of razor burn. Because they don't contain soaps, brushless creams are the best preshave products for men with dry skin.

Both Clinique and Aramis are now offering brushless shave creams. Aramis has the famous Aramis scent, while Clinique is fragrance-free. Much less expensive is Noxzema Medicated Brushless Shave Cream, which I find works just as well as the more expensive products.

Aerosol shave creams. Aerosols, the most popular preshave products, are similar to brushless creams in content. The reason they are so popular—many men have never thought to use another type of product—is because they are so convenient. Press the button on top of the can and you soon have your fingers full of preshave. Rub it on your face and you're ready to go.

Many men slap the foam on their face and start scraping right away. No good. Even if you use an aerosol cream for convenience, you should still let it sit on the face for two minutes after application to soften your beard. (To make your beard its softest, you should let any preshave product sit on the face for two minutes or so.)

Aerosol shave creams contain more alcohol than other preshaves and are therefore better for men with oily skin. If you have dry skin, a brushless shave cream is your best bet.

Today there are two types of aerosols: foam and the more recently developed gels. Gels may have one advantage: They can provide more even coverage and seem to hold the beard up better, which makes for a better shave.

If you like to use a menthol, lime- or lemon-scented shave cream, go ahead, but you should

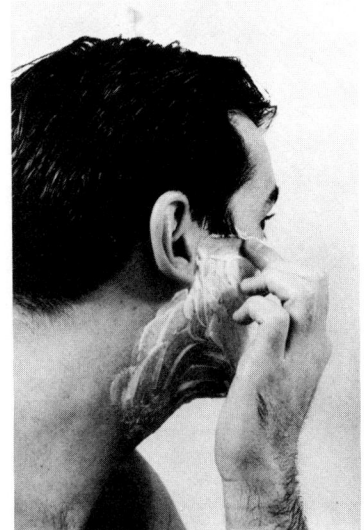

Make Your Shaving a Ritual.

Shaving should be something enjoyable, a pleasurable caring thing you do for yourself. Don't rush through your shave in the morning, worrying about being late to work. Think about your shaving and why you do it—to get the best-looking clean-shaven face you can. Shaving is a good time to look at and explore your face, so don't hurry through it. Look at yourself; notice your bone structure, the condition of your skin. Don't try to zip through the shave in a minute. You'll get a better shave.

A wet shave is the closest. Use an electric razor for touch-ups.

know that these added ingredients don't do much. "Medicated" shave creams sound nice, but they usually just contain more of the same healing ingredients found in other types of shave creams. Some of them will slightly numb the skin.

Many aerosol shave creams do a good job. Among them are Noxzema Medicated Shave, Barbasol, and Rise. All are good products at reasonable prices.

Step Four: Using Your Blades

With 75 million American men shaving once or more a day, the makers of shaving implements have tried their best to develop instruments to win the hearts and dollars of men. Well, they've done it. Today's razors are highly sophisticated.

You have a choice between single or twin-edge blades. Twin blades work, because in the act of shaving your whiskers are pulled up slightly from the skin by the first blade. By positioning a second blade about sixty-thousandths of an inch behind the first blade, the whiskers are cut before they have a chance to recede. Result: a much closer shave.

That is not to say that single blades don't work well. They do. Many men can't tell the difference between a double and single blade shave.

More important than whether you are using one or two blades is how sharp the blades are. A dull razor blade will cancel out all the water softening, preshave moisturizing, etc., that help make your shave the best possible. A sharp blade is a must.

One reason for making sure your blade is sharp is that a tiny layer of skin is always scraped off during shaving. If your blade is dull, this scraping becomes much more traumatic to your skin. It can result in

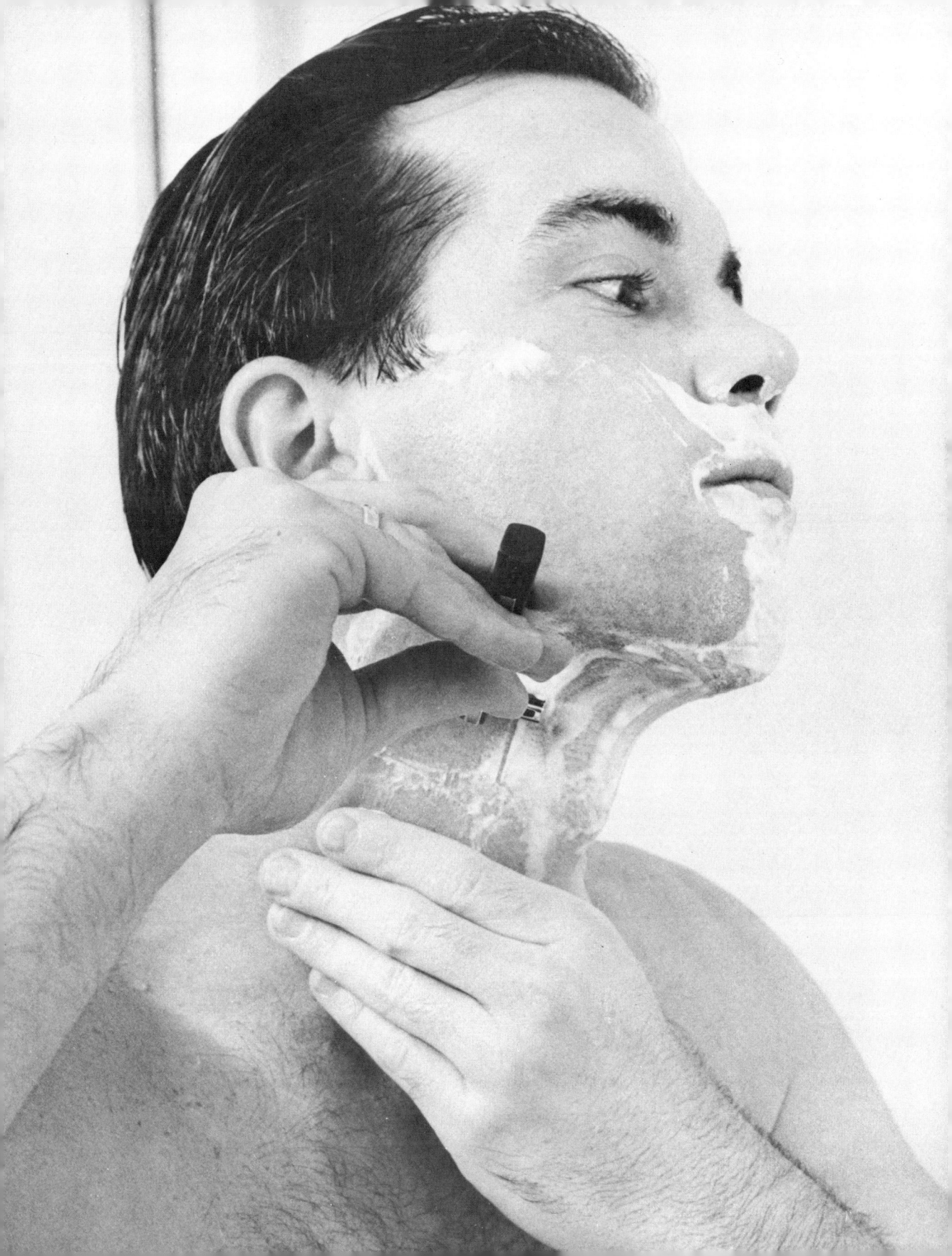

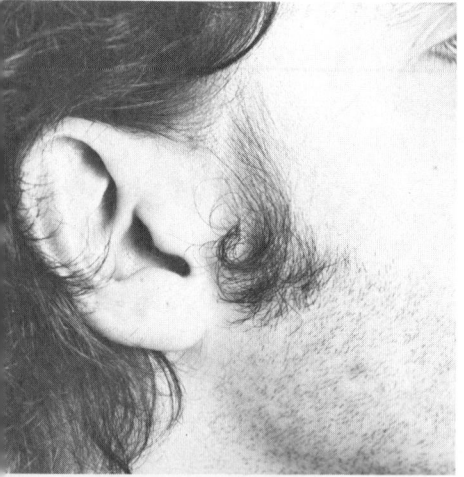

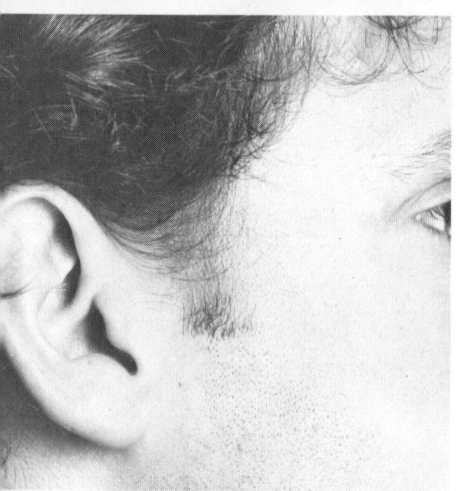

Your sideburns are visual arrows pointing to your cheekbones. When the sideburn is cut at bone level, your face gains a new structure. Feel your cheekbone. It has three surfaces: top, middle, and bottom. Ending your sideburns at the top of the cheekbone gives you a broader face; at the bottom of the cheekbone, a more narrow face. Pay special attention to the length of your sideburns when shaving.

skin that feels scratchy and looks blotchy.

My advice is to change your razor blade after every two shaves. The extra money is negligible if you consider shaving as a minor form of surgery, which is how you should view it.

Also, instead of wiping your blade with a tissue or towel to remove shave cream/whisker accumulations, rinse your blade under hot water before you begin to shave and after every few swipes across your face. Finish your shave by rinsing your blade for five to ten seconds before putting it away.

Once you are assured that you have a decent blade to work with, how to do you use it? There is a technique that virtually guarantees to rid you of shaving problems.

The secret: Shave *with the grain* of your beard. Somewhere along the line you may have learned that to get the absolutely, positively closest shave you should shave against the grain. True, this will give you a close shave. Unfortunately, it may also cause problems such as ingrown hairs, because shaving against the grain can cut whiskers below skin level. If this happens, watch out. The whiskers may grow into surrounding tissue instead of out the pore of the skin. Result: inflammation and possible infection.

The hair on your face has its own growth pattern, just as the hair on your head. For example, the whiskers on my face grow in a downward direction, while the hair on my neck grows up toward my chin. If you are unsure of the direction of your beard, you should let it grow for a day or two in order to see its direction.

To shave, start at your sideburns and wipe away the shave cream covering the bottom of the "burns" in order to get a good look at the cutting area. Remember, you want a clean edge to the sideburn so that it can be the best "arrow" possible in pointing to your cheekbones.

Your beard is denser around the chin and upper lip, so save these areas for last, allowing your shave cream to soften the beard for as long as possible. Shave with the grain. Pulling the skin taut may produce a closer shave, but if you have prepared your beard correctly, you should be able to skip this move.

Step Five: The Final Touches to a Perfect Shave

You have just de-whiskered your face. But in the process you have scraped off a thin layer of your face's skin, leaving it vulnerable to the elements. You must protect it.

What you do after you have finished shaving will in large part determine just how good your skin looks.

After your shave:

• Splash on warm water for a half minute, thoroughly rinsing all residues from the face.

• Next, turn the water to cool and splash your face some more. This will help close the pores of the skin, sealing in moisture.

• Now pat your face dry with a towel and apply a thin coat of moisturizer to the entire face and neck, locking in moisture and soothing skin that has been roughed up by shaving. When the moisturizer has dried to the touch you can splash on an after-shave lotion or cologne if you like, though a moisturizer provides a perfect ending to a shave in itself.

Paying closer attention to your shave is easy. And you'll get the best results possible.

To summarize how to get a great blade shave:

- **Soften your beard by washing with soap and hot water (taking a hot shower is even better).**
- **Use the right preshave product.**
- **Moisturize your skin.**
- **Use a sharp razor and shave with the grain of your beard.**
- **Rinse thoroughly.**
- **Close your pores and moisturize your skin again.**

The Electric Shave Routine

As with wet shaving, there's a right way to getting the best shave with an electric razor.

Preparing your beard for an electric shave requires using a preshave lotion. The lotion is an alcohol-based product that acts to dry up the oils on your skin and to make your whiskers stand straight up. Preshaves also contain additives that help the electric razor glide across the face. Unlike in wet shaving, your whiskers are most easily whisked away by an electric shaver if they are hard and stiff, making them easier to shear once they penetrate the shaver's heads.

If you have dry skin, you should not use a preshave lotion to set up your beard. It will dry your skin. For men with dry skin a preshave like Mennen Shave Talc is best, because it soaks up the oil on your skin without causing excessive dryness.

What type of electric razor is best? Consumer tests have shown the rotary-head design pioneered by Norelco to give the most comfortable shave.

Be sure to keep your electric razor clean by using the brush provided by the manufacturer after every shave. Also, have the blades in your electric razor replaced at the first sign of dullness. It's hard to imagine a worse routine for your skin than dragging a dull electric razor across your face every day.

When using an electric razor, be gentle. While it it tempting to grind the heads into your face in hopes of a closer cut, don't do it.

Manufacturers say the best way to use the shaver is to let *it* do the work. Run the shaver over your beard, in the direction of its growth. This will cut down on the chances that the shaver will hack your beard away in an uneven stubble.

After shaving with an electric razor, you may notice that the preshave lotion formulated to make your razor heads glide smoothly over your face is still there but feeling greasy. To rid your skin of the lotion, you should rinse your face with warm, then cool water, pat dry, and apply a moisturizer to smooth the skin.

Beards and Moustaches— How They Can Help Your Face

While a clean-shaven face is almost always correct, beards and moustaches take some thought. In many corporation situations, facial hair is frowned upon. In the United States military, except for the navy, there's no skipping the daily shave.

But if your business life allows you some leeway with your looks, consider what a beard or moustache can do for your face. Facial hair can work for you the way makeup works for women—it can play up your good features and very effectively disguise your weaknesses. It can balance heavy eyebrows, call attention to your smile, disguise thin lips, balance a receding hairline.

Forty-one percent of American men are now

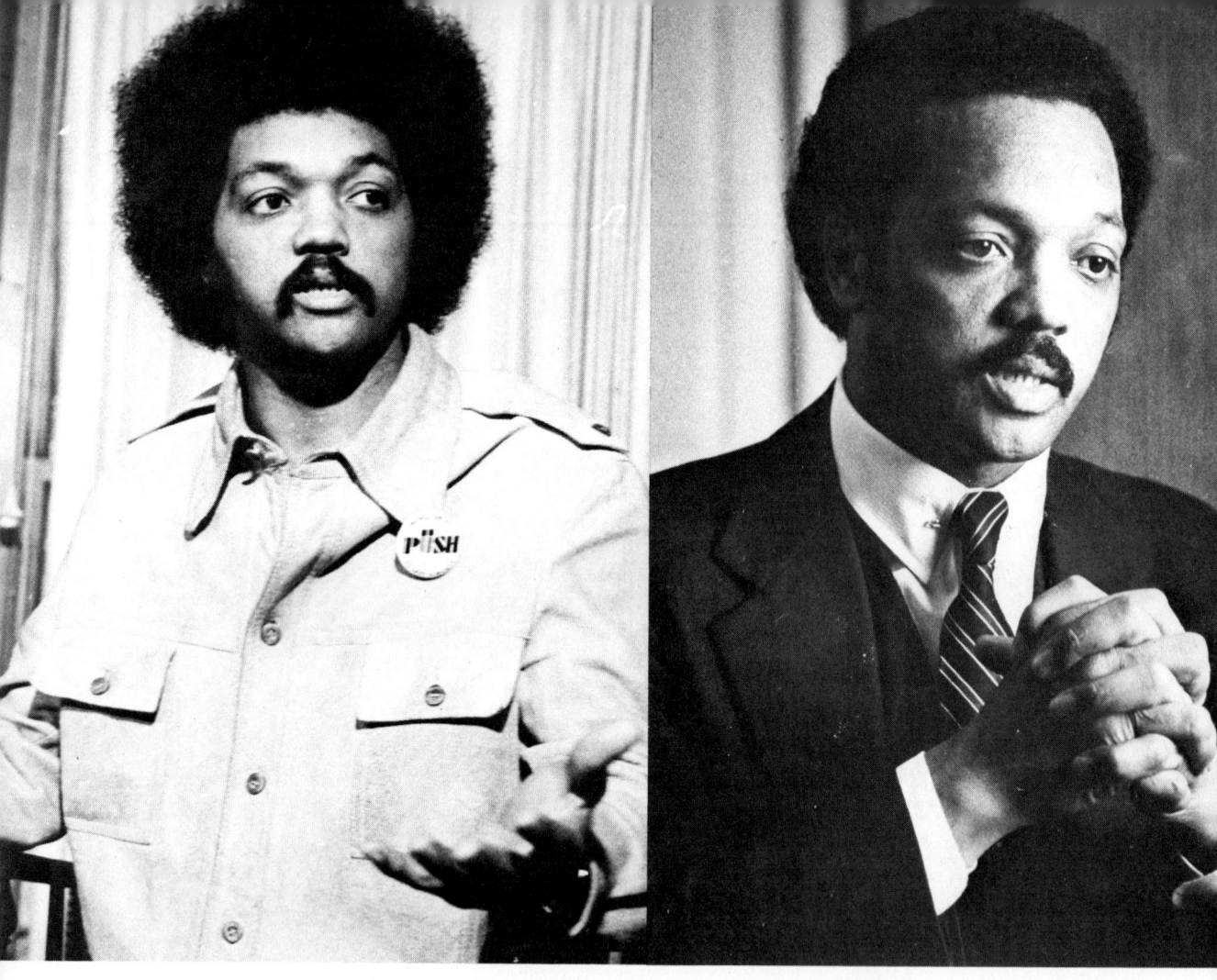

Jesse Jackson's very full Afro and Fu Manchu moustache were too radical for a presidential hopeful. Short hair and a well-trimmed moustache gave him the "power look" he was after. His well-groomed appearance now projects authority at any level of business or politics and gives new strength to his message.

sporting some kind of facial hair, whether it's a Tom Selleck moustache or a full Kris Kristofferson beard. So the subject of whether or not to grow a beard or moustache is a visible option for most men.

Moustaches

• A moustache will generally make a young man look older and add more character to an older man's face. If you have always had a baby face and feel you might command more respect with a moustache, then by all means give it a try.

- Moustaches can help a thin upper lip by filling in the area between the bottom of the nose and the mouth, strengthening this section of your face while concealing your lip.

- If a man has a large forehead, it tends to dominate his face. Growing a moustache will draw the eye down toward the center of the face for a more balanced look.

- If your hair is thinning, a moustache or beard will draw attention away from your thinning hair and down your face. It's certainly worth a try. If it doesn't work, shave it off. (Give it four weeks before you make a final judgment.)

- If you have close-set eyes, a moustache may not be for you. Remember, a moustache brings attention to the *center* of the face. If you have close-set eyes, you want to bring the attention *outward* instead.

- If you have a large nose, growing a moustache will bring the balance of your face more into proportion. From the side view, a moustache will "fill in," adding thickness to the area under your nose, making the jump from the nose to the mouth less large.

How to Trim Your Moustache

While dozens of moustache shapes have come and gone, today the best moustache is the simplest one. It is the "bottom trimmed" moustache, in which the hair between the nose and mouth is left to grow and then clipped along the line of the top lip.

This type of moustache is masculine, gives a powerful look, and doesn't require elaborate trimming or shaping. Today, such styles as Fu Manchu's

Political aspirations call for a "power look."

and walrus moustaches look too contrived.

To trim your moustache:

- Work with a dry moustache. Hair shrinks when dry, stretches when wet. If you cut your moustache when it's wet, it may be too short when it dries.

- With a small-toothed comb, comb the hair down toward your lips. Use the top of your lip as a guide, and start cutting from the middle of the moustache, cutting first to one side and then the other. This will give you a more even trim.

- Now comb the moustache to either side, and trim any stray hairs and the outer edges. **The edges of a moustache shouldn't extend more than a quarter inch outside the lips. Your smile lines are the best guide to where to trim.**

- You don't have to shave or trim the top of your moustache. Let it grow all the way up to your nose. Skinny moustaches only look good on character actors in the movies (Clark Gable).

When Jesse Jackson was running for president, John Weitz, the men's wear designer, suggested that Jackson trim his Fu Manchu moustache because it made him look sinister. Jackson took the advice and he did look better, demonstrating that a neat shape and proper trimming are the keys to good-looking facial hair. ("Page Six" of the *New York Post* featured the "before" and "after" photos.)

Beards

Like moustaches, beards draw attention to themselves, camouflaging unflattering facial features. The right beard can bring a man's face into proportion and adds a look of strength and virility to the face. It can give a man the look of authority.

In ancient Egypt, the higher a man's rank, the longer his beard; likewise in Persia and Assyria. Slaves were forced to shave.

But leave the shapes seen in history books and gladiator movies to the past. And avoid the Mephistopheles goatee. There are few faces that can take its rather theatrical look.

Today's beard is well trimmed and well shaped. It's clean and soft, not scratchy. It's manageable and easy to care for. Here are some of the benefits of beards:

- They counterbalance a receding hairline. When the hair on your head starts to go, a beard can add a missing dimension to your face. Remember to keep the beard fairly short, or you will reverse the balance of your face, becoming bottom heavy.
- They make a craggy face much less forboding. Very strong cheekbones on a too slim face can be balanced and softened by a full beard—one left to grow naturally on the cheeks rather than sculpted with a razor.
- They give the appearance of solid bone structure to a weak chin. You'll want a beard that gives the visual impression of bulk and sharp definition to the lower face.
- They camouflage sharp, pointy chins. A full beard will visually double the size of your chin, make it look less sharp.
- They add some color and interest to a face with winter-pale skin. Your facial structure will determine the shape of the growth, but the most important thing is that you get some color onto the face.
- They widen the too narrow face. Here, a

A scruffy beard detracts from your face. Keep it trimmed.

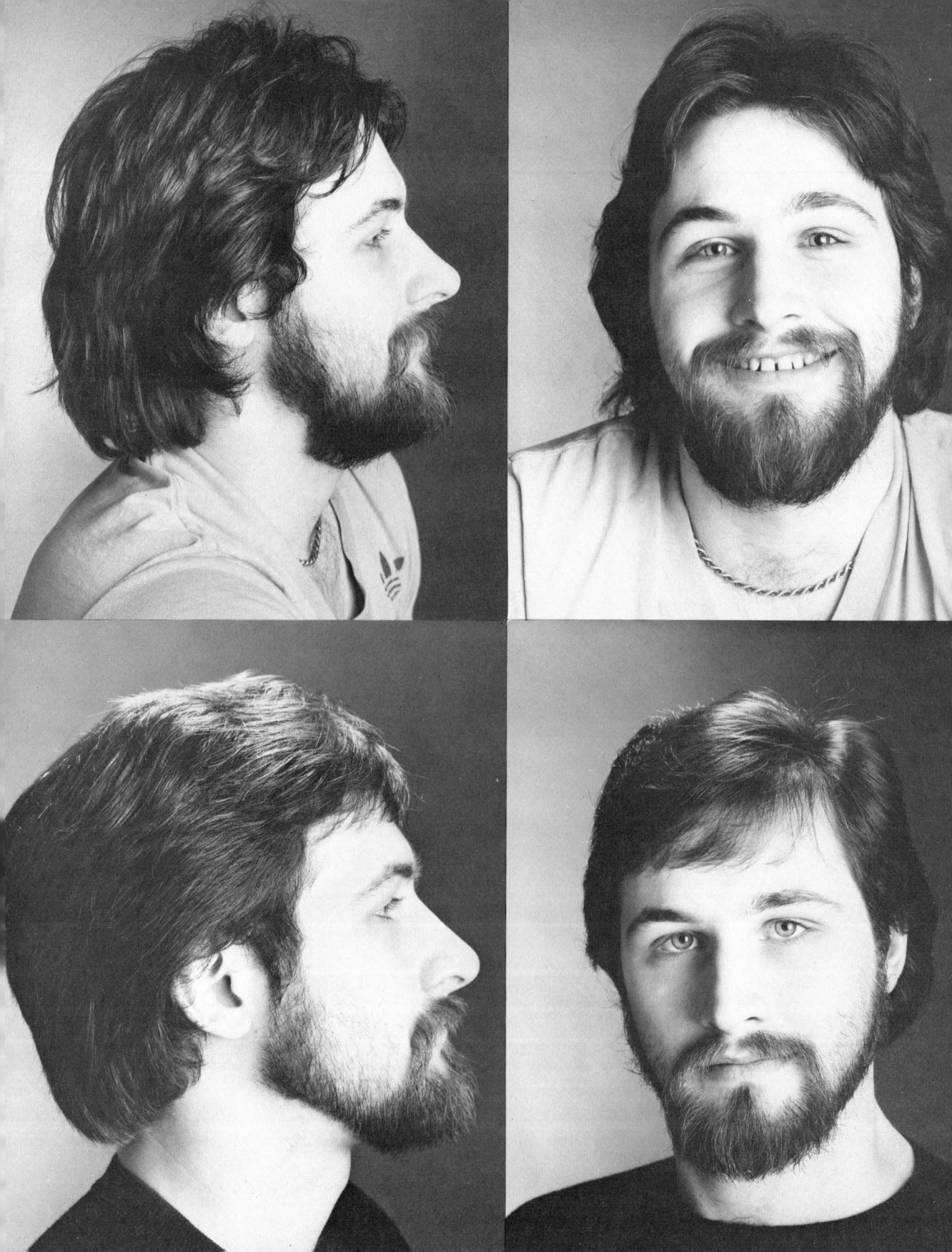

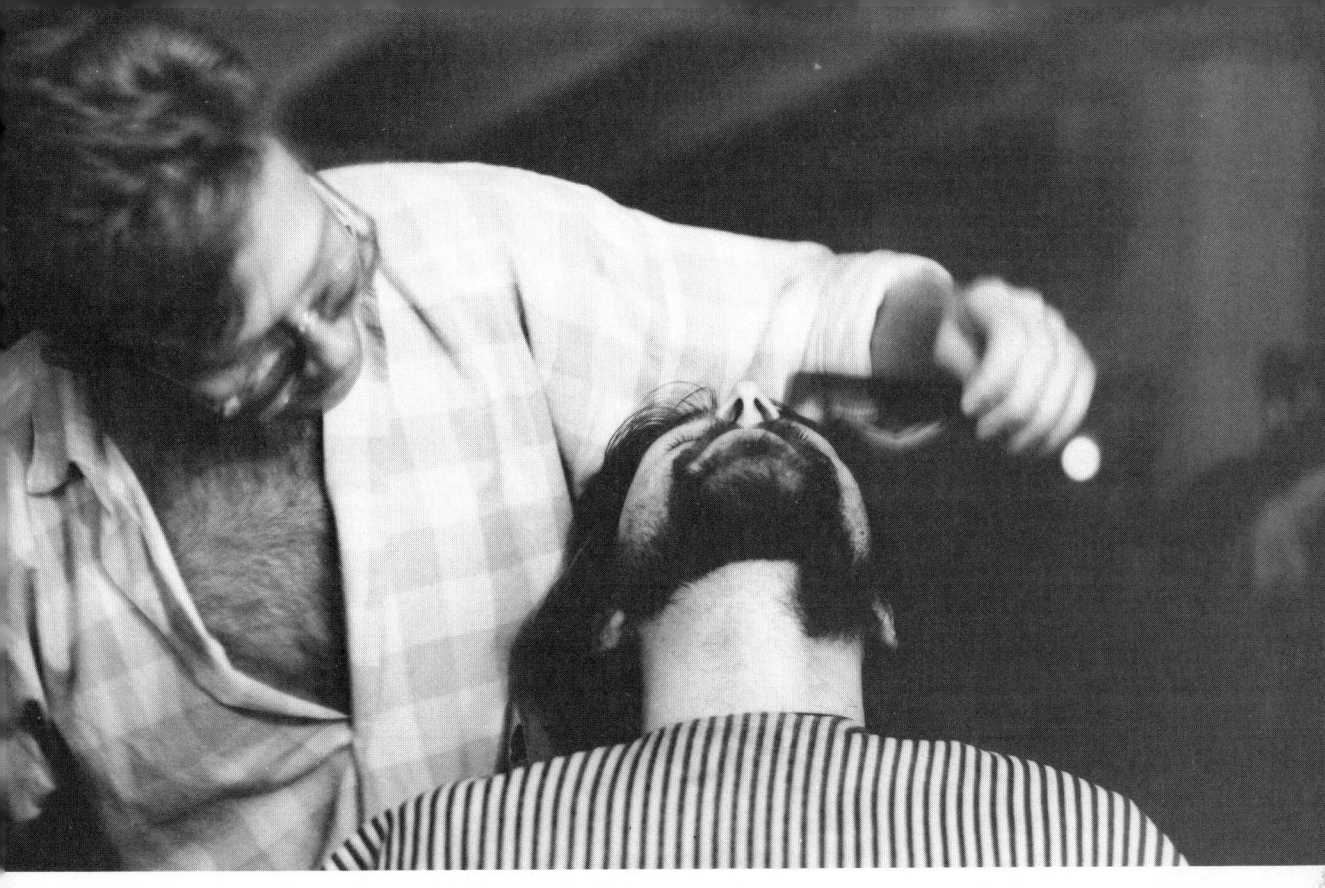

Peter

A design line gives your beard shape.

Peter's beard was overgrown and had no definite shape. The absence of a design line at the neck made his face look fuller. A U-shaped design line removed bulk from under the chin, making his jawline appear stronger. I encouraged Peter to stop shaving his cheek area, fill in his beard, and avoid the skimpy chin-strap look.

beard gives you a strong horizontal line. If you feel your face is too thin, a beard will add a look of power and solidity while visually widening your face.

● They can mask disfigurations, such as acne pits or scars from accidents.

How to Grow Your Beard

Nothing could be easier than growing a beard. You just stop shaving.

However, you won't be the proud owner of a fine beard for quite some time. The time it takes to foster enough hair to see what's what varies from man to man. Plan on looking ragged for at least three weeks, so the best time to start is during your vacation.

During the first weeks, your face may itch. You'll endure this period, all the while making sure to keep your face clean.

While it would be natural to assume that your beard would be the same color as the hair on your head, this is seldom the case. You'll have to wait and see what color the hair grows in to see if you like it. You may find it comes in a very interesting shading of gray hairs, such as Kris Kristofferson's or that of "60 Minutes" correspondent Ed Bradley.

Shaping Your Beard for Maximum Effect

After four weeks, your beard should reach a full enough growth so you will be able to see what it finally will look like—where the hair grows fullest, where the thin spots are. Just as with the hair on your head, your beard may have a thin spot.

You are now ready to shape your beard. Here's

how to design it, to make sure it does what you want it to and relates to your facial features.

There are two prcedures for keeping a beard in top shape:

- Keeping the edges of the beard looking clean and in a shape that complements your face
- Keeping the beard itself trimmed in a neat, well-groomed manner

The edges forming the outline of the beard determine how the beard relates to your facial features. Here is how to make the most of the edges of your beard:

- Look into the bathroom mirror, lift your chin, and observe your jawline. You will see that your jaw is curved. This curve is the shape you should create in your *neck design line,* the bottom line of your beard. It will be in a slight U-shape, never straight. The exception: If you have a thin face, a square neck design line will make your face look heavier.

- To create your design line, follow the directions above for shaving when wetting and lathering the hair under your chin. Before you take a razor to the beard, wipe off the shaving cream to get a clear view of where you will be cutting. The design line should be about a half inch below the outside edges of the jawline.

The other edge you will have to maintain is the top edge of the beard, on your cheeks. You are free to leave the top line natural for a full beard, which is the best look—unless you have a hairy face or would like to make your jaw look more square.

To give a stronger shape to the jaw, a design line for the top of the beard would descend from the sideburn and reach farther down into the beard

A moustache or beard will make you look older.

where the jaw curves forward. This will also widen the bottom portion of your face—good for men with heart-shaped faces and/or pointed chins.

Once your design lines are established, shave them three times a week to keep the edges neat.

Once you have established the boundaries of your beard, what's the best way to keep the beard itself in top form? I suggest growing a beard a maximum of one inch in length for a clean trim look. The quickest, surest way to keep your beard groomed is with a set of professional barber clippers. Men often fiddle with a comb and a pair of scissors to trim their beards, but the results are extremely difficult to gauge.

Clippers are an easy way to keep your beard neat. They range in price from $15 and up. They come equipped with a separate set of guard attachments, which fit over the end of the clippers. The attachments range in size from a quarter inch to an inch. Simply attach the right size guard on the clippers and run them over your beard in the direction of its growth. A biweekly groom with clippers will maintain your beard at just the right length, whatever that length is up to an inch.

Use scissors to clean up the edges of your beard around the ears and the lip. Clippers can be used without the guard attachment on the design line of your neck.

You should wash your beard or moustache every time you wash your hair, and you should use the same shampoo. It's a good idea to use a conditioner on your facial hair (the same one you use on your head) once a week to keep it soft and shiny.

After shampooing your facial hair, comb it with a wide-toothed comb to rid it of tangles. Then brush the beard with short strokes in the direction that you would like it to lie.

A toothbrush with firm bristles makes a good beard brush, or you can buy a brush especially made for the purpose. Whatever brush you use, you should make sure the entire depth of your beard is groomed, not just the top hairs.

Treating your beard to its own grooming regimen will pay off with a beard that is luxurious to the touch and the eyes. Is there any other beard worth having?

Another New You

Many men grow facial hair when they are in college to look older. No problem with that.

Some men keep their facial hair longer than is needed. If you've been wearing your facial hair for more than a few years, I have a suggestion: Shave it off.

That's right, shave it. It will always grow back if you decide that you need it, but you may discover that your face has changed to the point that you no longer want your facial hair. Also, after reading this book you may decide that a new haircut can remedy the problems that caused you to grow a beard or moustache.

Here's how to proceed:

● If you have a pair of barber's clippers, use *no* guard and cut hair off close.

● If you don't have clippers, use scissors to trim as much of the hair on your face as possible.

● Then hop in the shower and follow the directions for getting a great shave.

● Once shaved, go back to the beginning of this book and start over in finding a new look for the "new" you.

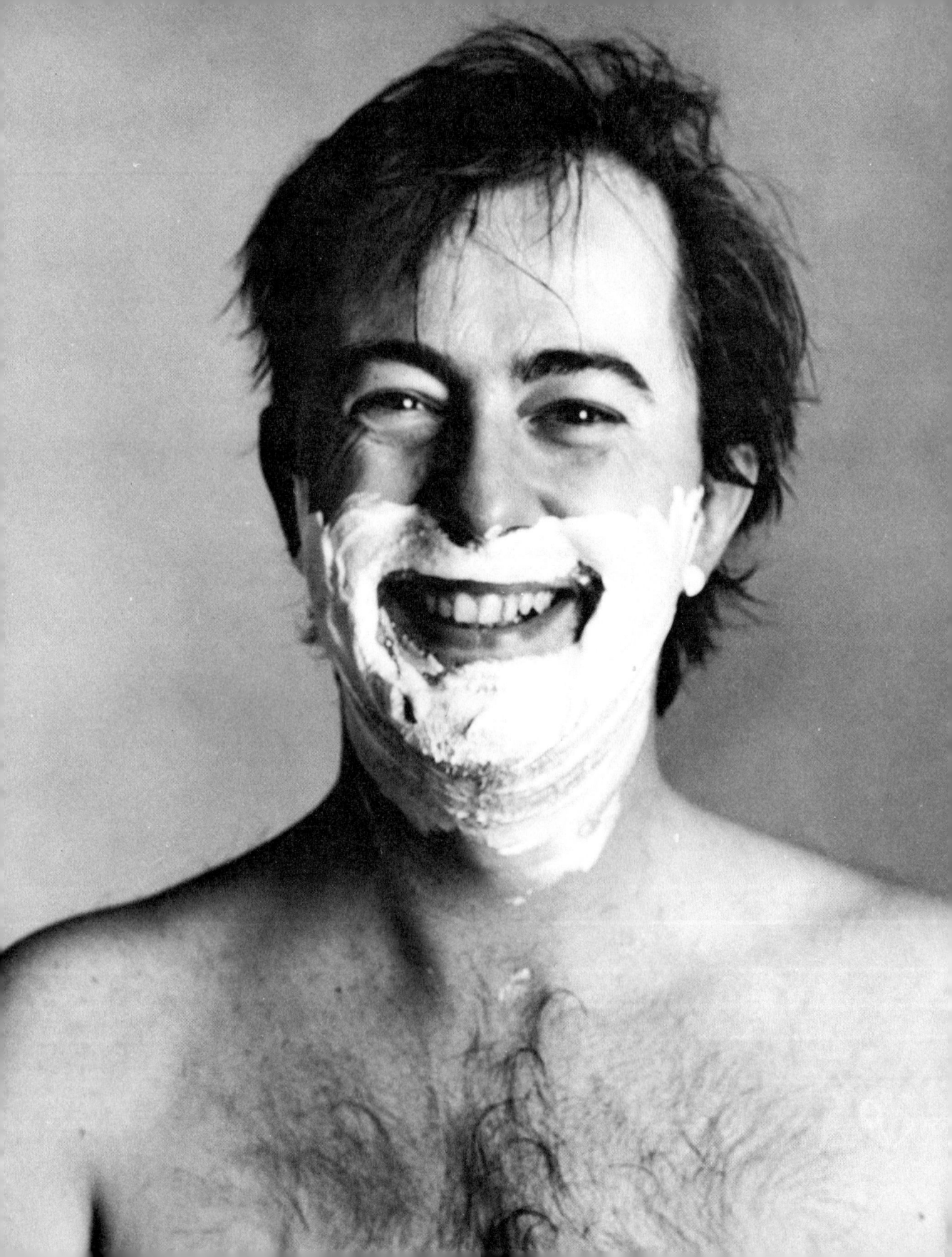

Interview with Guy

I hadn't shaved more than my neck for thirteen years when I met George Roberson in New York. The growth on my jaw dated back to January 1971. I was nineteen; it was the post-Hippie era, and everyone else in the Vermont college where I was a sophomore was growing a beard—well, everyone who could—so it was natural for me to follow suit. I'd never really questioned having a beard in the thirteen years I let it take over; I often forgot that I had one. It was part of me.

George decided it didn't *have* to be. "You'd make a perfect makeover," he told me, focusing his expert eye on my hirsute jaw. (Not the most flattering comment I've ever received, but he was the expert.)

"You mean I *do* have a chin?" I asked him incredulously.

"Well, *something's* under there," he replied. "Want to find out what?"

I wasn't sure that I did, but what did I know? Maybe there was a Robert Redford screaming to get out. I drummed up courage and said okay.

Two weeks later. Look at the second picture. It says more than I could, except that it doesn't show the utter terror I felt beneath that hysterical smile.

Five minutes after that. Good god, there was *air* out there. I could feel it on my face. My face! I had one! I looked into the mirror and said, "Excuse me," when suddenly I realized that the reflected image staring back at me *was* me. The old self was gone, completely gone. I didn't even recognize my eyes. They seemed larger. *This* was me? You don't

Out from under a beard after years

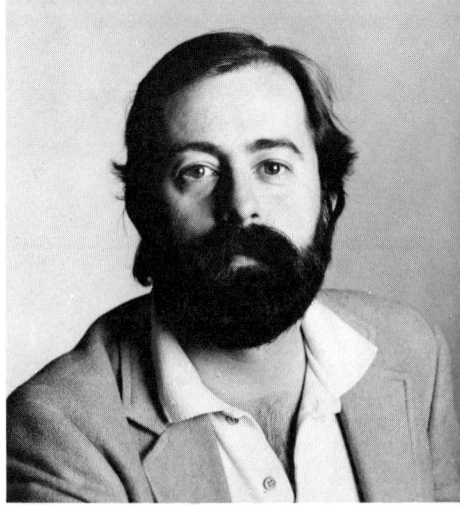

Guy looked like his "before" shot for at least ten years. He rarely altered his appearance. We decided to go for a clean sweep. You can see Guy's anxiety in the shaving cream photo. *Voilà!* Our final look: clean-shaven after thirteen years. He rediscovered his hidden bone structure. The short, neat beard gives his jaw shape, and the wisp of forehead hair gives his eyes intensity.

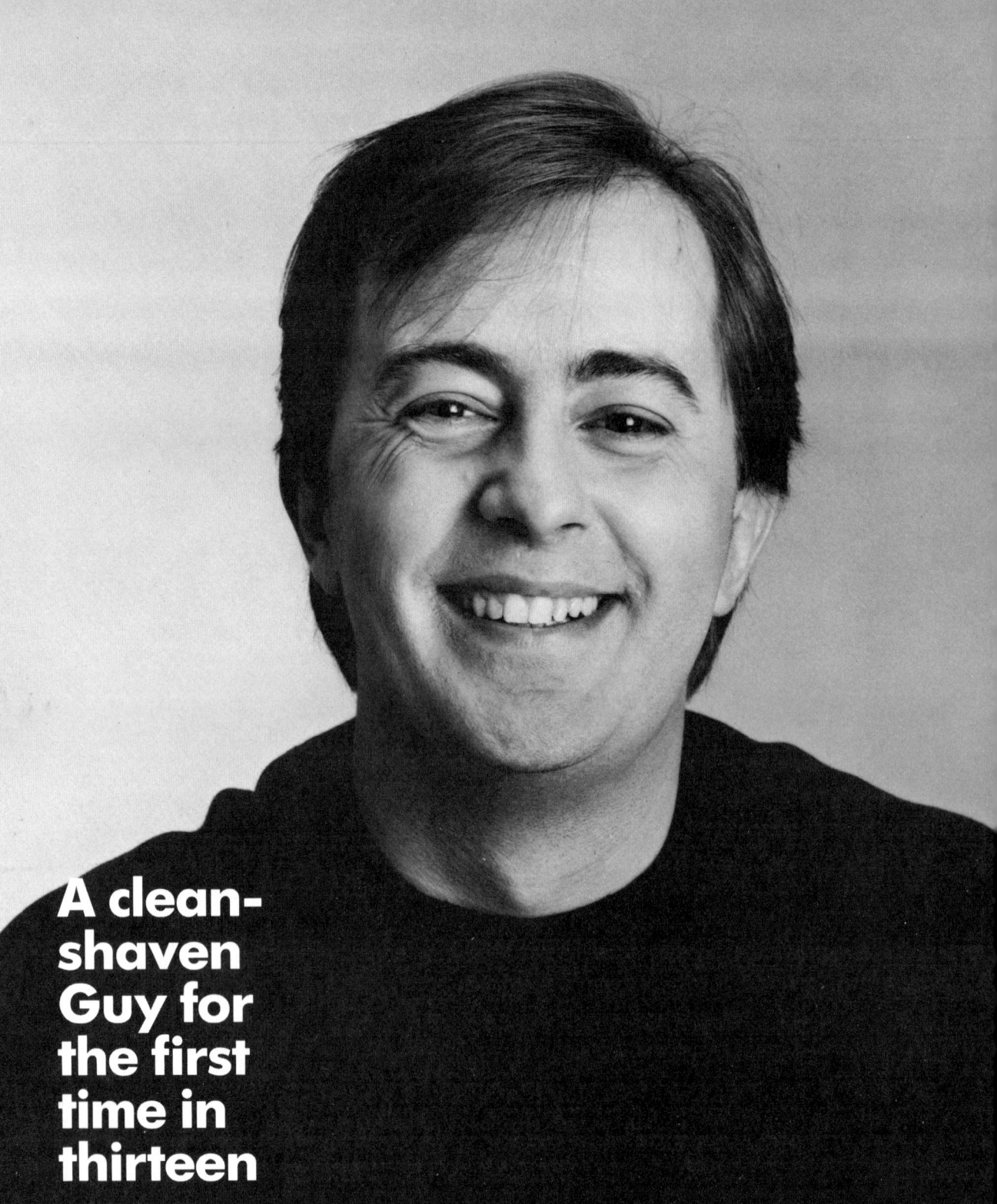

A clean-shaven Guy for the first time in thirteen years

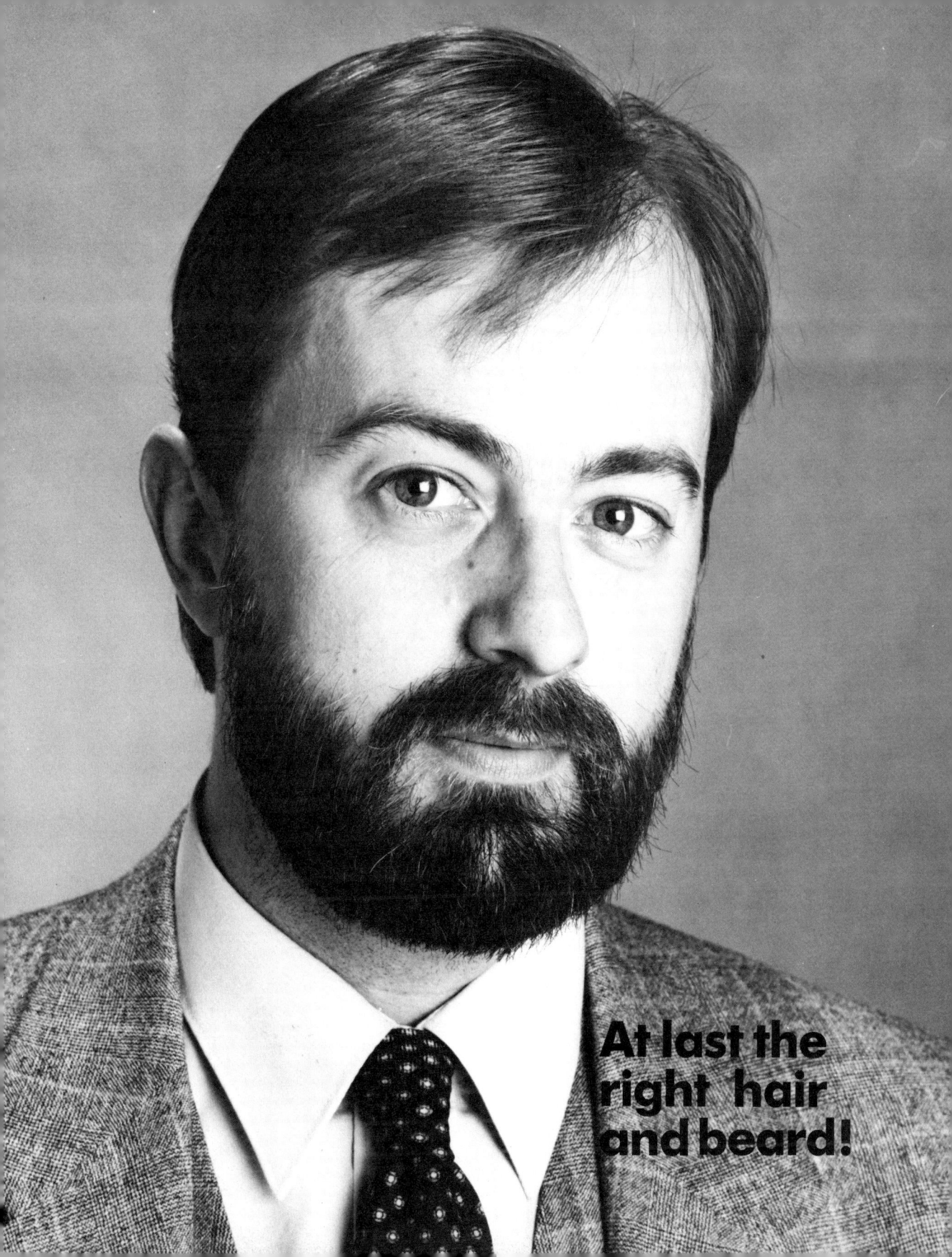

At last the
right hair
and beard!

know the meaning of confusion until you've lost a thirteen-year-old beard.

I decided to foist the new me on my parents and took a train that weekend out to their home in Long Island. I knocked on the door. When my mother opened it, she had no idea who I was. Neither, for the next week that I shaved, did I.

Rebirth. Not having a beard was at least fascinating, but I had to admit (George eventually did, too) that a beard *did* do something for me. I'd learned a few lessons, however: My face does have a shape; I do have eyes; I do, after a fashion, have a chin. (I even have lips.) The task, said George, was to make whatever was good about those details stand out. The beard came back (although this time with six gray hairs in it—trauma) and George gave me another going-over. He'd known all along what I hadn't, that by seeing my face and understanding its "architecture," I'd know how to use my beard to frame it. He's actually gotten me to trim the damned thing.

And for the first time in thirteen years, my smile isn't lost under my moustache. (Thank you, Mr. Roberson.)

Should you grow facial hair? There are certainly plenty of sound reasons to consider this option when coming up with a look for yourself. Whether you need a beard or moustache to give you a psychological boost or to strengthen specific facial features, it can't hurt to try the look of hair on your face. Like any other hair option, the only thing that's permanent about facial hair is your satisfaction in finding the look that's right for you.

9.

WAVES

A Wave Can Bring New Possibilities to Your Hairstyle

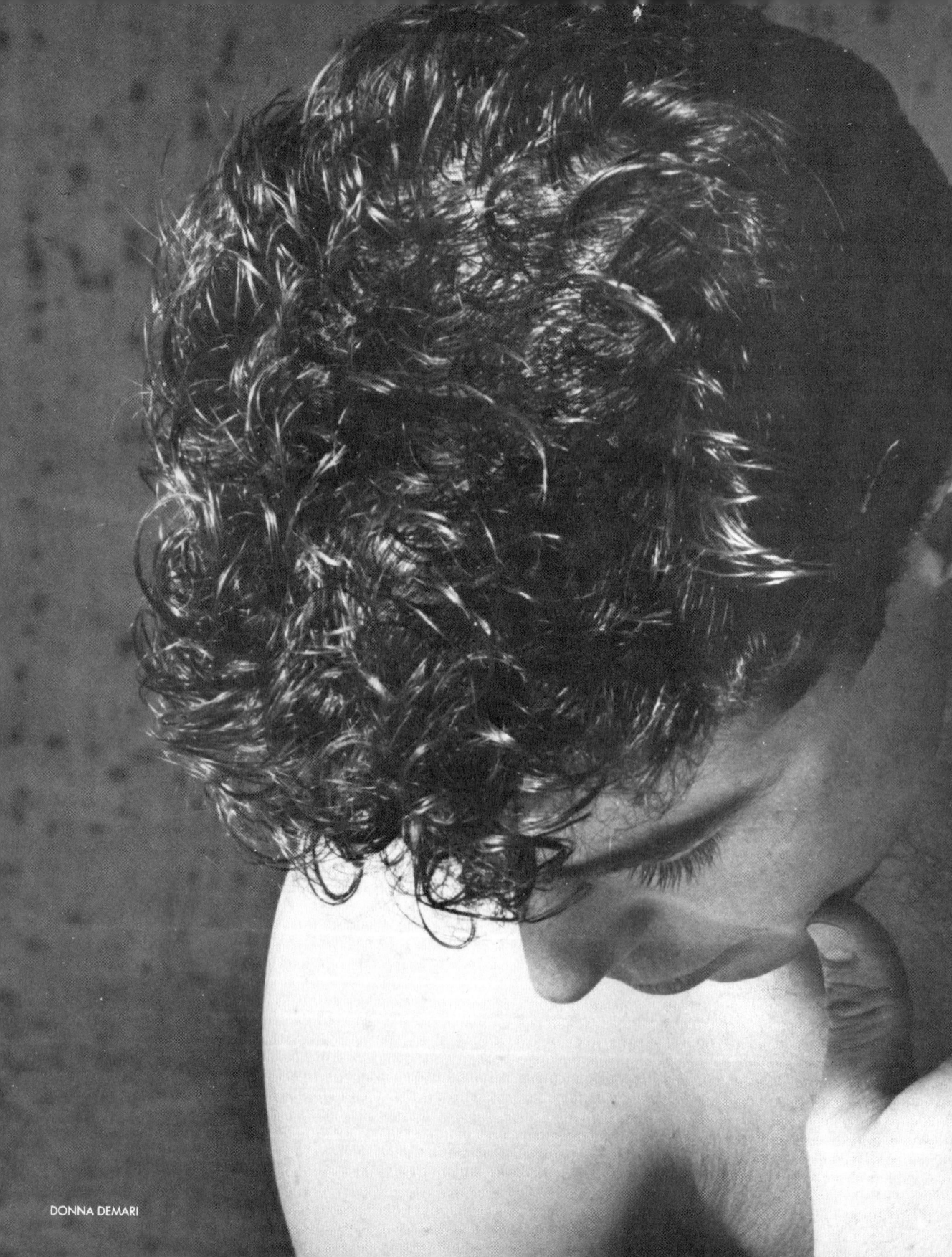

What a Wave Can Do to Boost Your Image

A permanent wave is one of the most effective techniques for making your hair do what *you* want it to do. It can literally change the character of your hair, giving it new body, shape, and movement.

Most of us, when we think of permanents, think of curls. More unfavorably, we remember the heads full of frizz that were signatures of free-thinking hair stylists of the '60s and '70s. That image is not only outdated, it's misleading. A permanent will not produce a headfull of frizz unless that is what you aim for.

Waving is a more accurate way of describing the permanent process. It hints at the fact that you can control the straightness, curliness, and texture of your hair to a fine degree. You can make limp hair thicker and curlier. You can straighten too-curly hair. You can take your hair through the whole range of thin to thick, straight to curly, fine-tuning it to get exactly the look you want.

Here are some of the basic problems a wave could solve for you:

- It can *lift* hair that looks flat on your head, by adding more body.
- It can *add bulk* to hair that is thinning.
- It can *unify* the hair on your head, making it all straight or all wavy.

- It can make your hair *hold a style* and a shape that it would not hold naturally.
- It can *revive* a wave that disappeared with the years.
- It can give you the *option* of a seasonal change in hair, say straighter in summer, curlier in winter.

How Waves Work

Waving has become a very sophisticated process. So I advise having your first permanents done by a professional. Your stylist can evaluate the condition of your hair. He knows all the products available and which is the best for you. Most important, he'll time the process accurately, a tricky operation for the amateur to do.

When you wave your hair, you actually change the hair's natural structure chemically. The structure of each hair shaft on your head is determined by the chemical bonds within the inner core of the shaft, the cortex. The waving chemicals break down the chemical bonds within the hair and rebuild them according to your wishes, going from straight to curly or vice versa.

A word of reassurance: Chemical processing will not cause you to lose hair or affect new growth of hair. But you cannot reverse the wave process—hence the word *permanent* to describe this technique of breaking down and rebuilding the hair structure. Of course, since new hair growth is untouched by the waving process, if you don't like your waved hair, you simply grow new hair and cut off the processed part.

The Wave Procedure

Waves are usually categorized as "warm waves,"

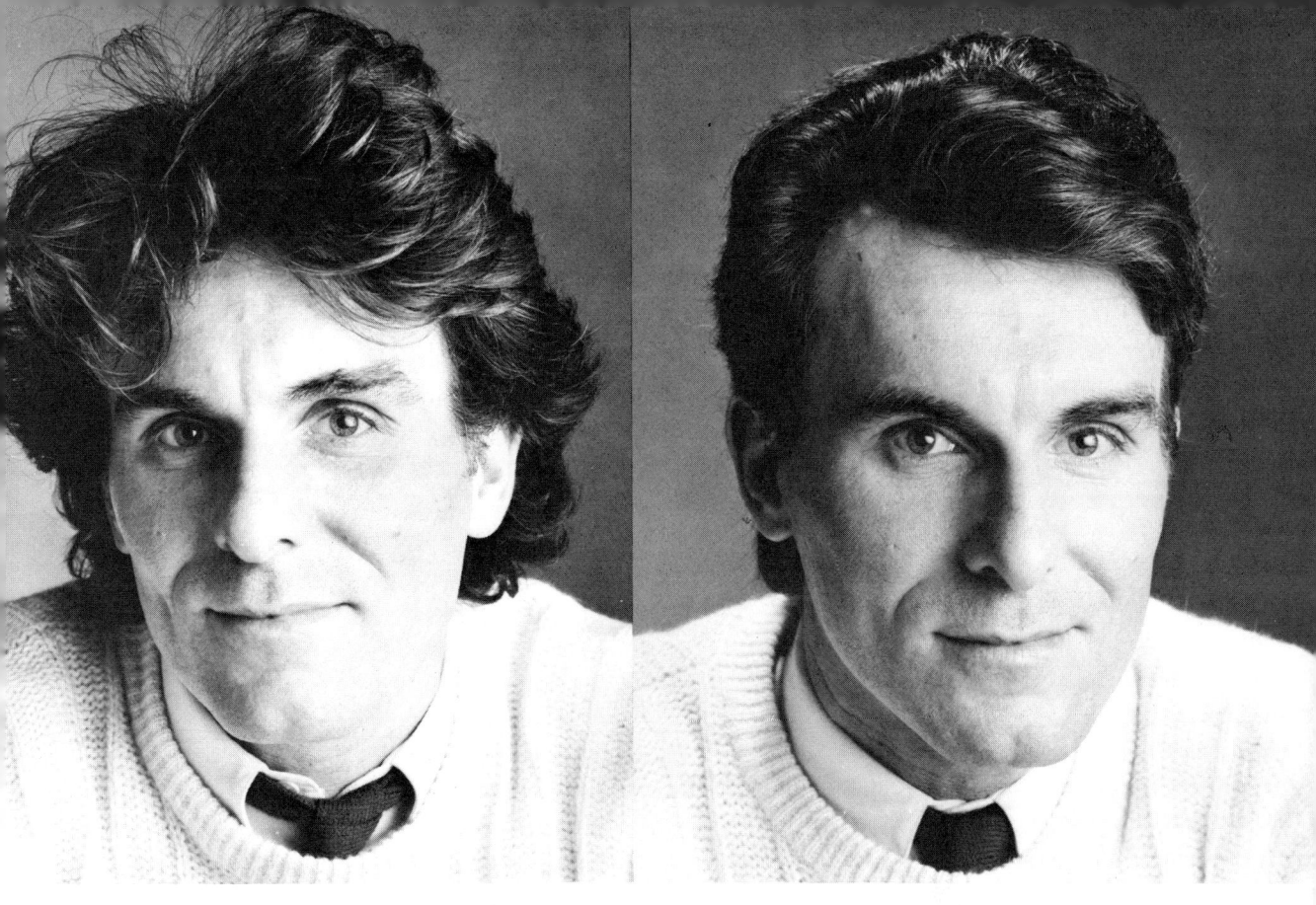

Albert

Medium-length wavy hair can be over-powering.

Wavy hair can be fun, rock 'n' roll, a bit of a mess. That's great when you want to project that image, but at times you need to look more polished. Hair worn close to the head is usually accepted as more professional. A medium-length cut can be smoothed quickly with a blow dryer for an instant change.

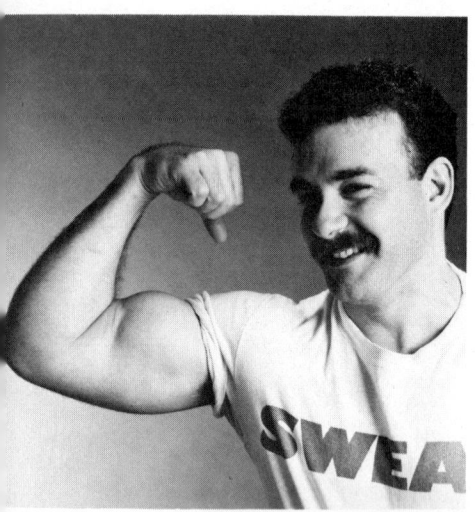

Tom has wavy, curly hair. Weekly deep-conditioning keeps it soft and shiny.

which use heat to help set the curl, and "cold waves," which use no heat but stronger chemicals.

Risky business: The waving kits you can buy for home use are cold waves. Don't bother with them. Have a professional give you a warm wave. It's less hard on your hair, and it's best to let a pro judge how long the different solutions should be left on. Timing is critical. If the waving solution is left on too long, you may ruin the condition of your hair and you also may get more curl than you planned. Once again, go with a pro.

With the warm wave procedure, the hair to be waved—your entire head or a section, maybe just the top—is first shampooed, then the damp hair is wound onto perm rods. The larger the diameter of the rod, the bigger the curl. If your hair only needs a bit of added height or lift, you'll get the largest rod for the length of your hair. If you want more wave or curl, you'll be waved with smaller rods. The bigger the perm rod, the larger the wave. The smaller the rod, the tighter the wave.

After all the hair is wound onto rods, your hairline is wrapped in cotton and the processing solution is applied to the hair. A plastic bag goes over your hair and you go under the dryer for five to twenty minutes so the heat can help the chemicals penetrate the hair shaft.

After the length of time determined by your stylist, you emerge from the dryer and he rinses out the solution. He will blot your still-rolled hair with a towel, apply fresh cotton and then another solution, the neutralizer, which locks in the new shape of the hair. After another five to ten minutes, the rods are removed and the solution is rinsed out of the hair.

If you like the result, you'll want to repeat the process in two to four months. Remember, every haircut cuts off some of the chemically waved hair. If you have thick straight hair and you wear a curly wave, you'll get a quick line of demarcation as soon as the new hair grows in. You'll be able to see the difference between the new growth and the processed hair. Also, the new growth, which is straight, will lack the curl support at the roots that the processing gives and may cause the hair to fall flatter to the head. It won't have the same lift as when it was originally waved. In order to maintain a style, you may then need to alter the way you wear your hair by parting it.

If you have a looser wave put into the hair, the new growth line won't show as much. You can go longer without having to get a new wave put in the hair.

As a general rule, the more drastic the change in your hair—for instance, going from straight to very curly—the more often you'll need to repeat the wave. A partial wave to blend in the top or sides of your head with the rest of your naturally curly hair would require less frequent touch-ups. The more similarity between your natural hair and your waved hair, the longer the waved look will last.

How Curly to Go

Curly waves. Here's a good look to disguise thinning or receding hair. The overall curliness can camouflage the hairline. In addition, curly hair takes up more space, looks bulkier because air space is created between individual hair shafts. It also softens a man's appearance, playing down bold

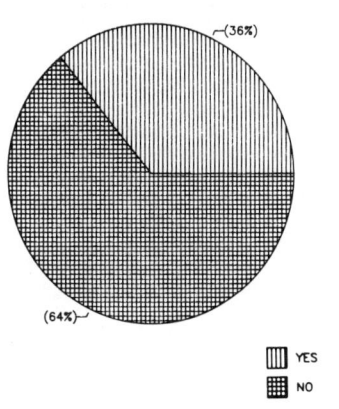

HAVE YOU EVER HAD A PERM OR A WAVE?

(36%)

(64%)

▥ YES
▦ NO

The slightest wave gives hair maximum effect.

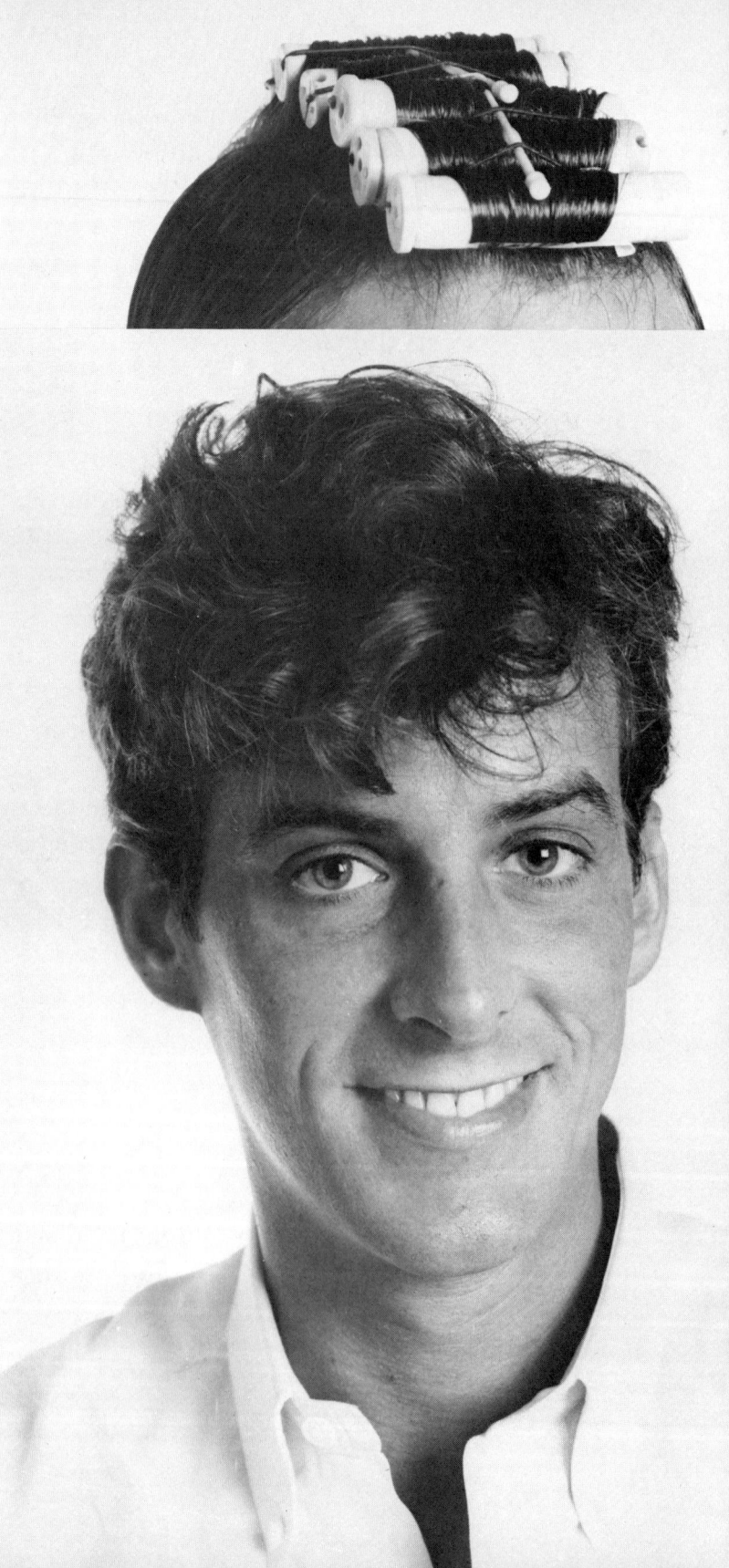

Stewart likes to wear his hair long on top and short at the sides. His slightly wavy hair went flat from the extra weight on top. A heat-activated body wave was applied only to the top of his head. The fuller, wavy hair adds softness to Stewart's oblong face. Easy. Soft. Believable. He'll rewave every four months.

facial features. It can work for softer features, too, creating an overall pleasant appearance.

Curly hair is easy to maintain. You can comb it with your fingers after a shower. And it's versatile. Leave it as is—totally free, natural, casual. Shape it with a hair groomer, and part it on the side for a more elegant, controlled look, suitable to any business situation.

Semicurly waves. When curls are very large, they become waves, hair with an undulating shape. Semicurly waves produce curls so large that, when hair is combed or brushed, they fall into rippling lines within the hair.

You should have a medium or thick amount of hair for a semicurly wave. It will help tame coarse, unruly hair that needs more than a good cut to behave. The wave would even out the curliness in the hair, making it more manageable. Then it could be styled to make the most of your facial features.

Like a tan, a wave in the hair makes almost any man look better. It has movement. This type of wave has the most versatile styling possibilities. It can adapt to sporty or elegant looks, depending upon how your groom it. You can use your fingers, a wide-toothed comb, or a brush with widely spaced bristles to shape your hair casually. Or keep it well under control with an oily hair dressing like VO5 or Brylcreem.

The body wave. This is the mildest and most useful wave for men. It adds extra texture to the hair without waves or curls. If you have the kind of hair that lies flat on your head, that flies away in a breeze, a body wave will add texture and holding power to your hair.

Body waves are useful for adjusting the *proportions* of your hairstyle, adding fullness to the hair on the sides of your head to help frame your face effectively, adding more bulk on the top of your head to even out the proportions of a triangular face. If you need extra volume in just *one* spot, consider a body wave.

Partial body waves can help if the hair on top of your head is thinning and lying flat, looking out of proportion to the rest of your hair. A wave put in the flat area at the top will fluff it up to match the volume of the hair at the sides and back.

A body wave helps hair hold its shape by giving it more *texture*. More texture equals greater holding power. With the added volume a body wave gives to your hair, you will now be able to blow-dry your fine hair into a shape it will hold. Simply apply a good hair spray or setting lotion after you blow-dry and your style will stay put.

Straightening waves. The last type of wave does exactly what it says. Instead of adding curl, it eases curly hair into a straighter shape. The process is the same as for any other wave, except for the size of the rods. Very large rods are used to stretch the curl out of the hair.

From the above you can see that waves may be able to make your hair do what proper cutting and maintenance can't. Here are some other ways that waves can solve specific problems.

• Waves can help you cope with different hair formations.

Different hair formations on the same head can look odd. For example, if you have wavy or curly hair all over your head except on top, where the hair is straight, a partial wave on the straight hair

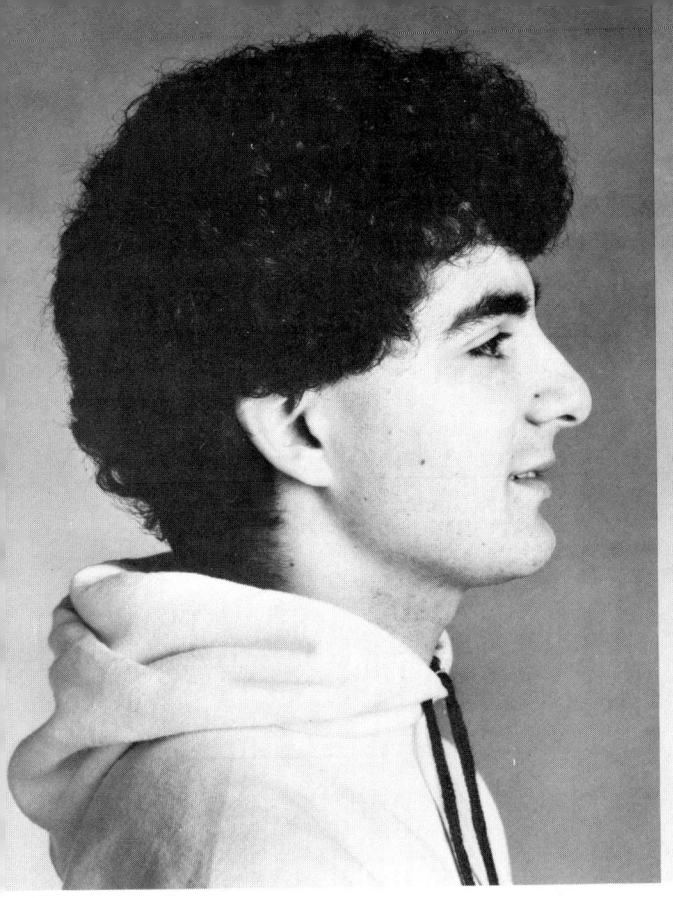
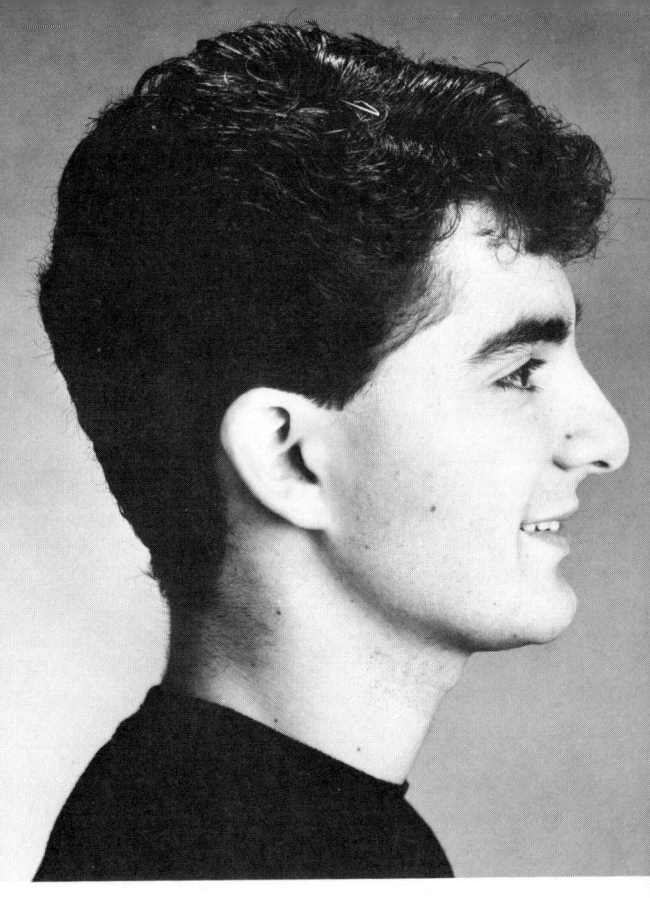

Jeff

Curly hair out of hand, in the wrong shape

Eighty percent of all men look best with a square-shaped haircut. Jeff is a case in point. Close hair on the sides of the head always attracts more attention to the eyes. Curly hair like Jeff's tends to grow full instead of long, making his head look bigger and his bone structure less defined. Weekly conditioning makes curly hair shiny and soft instead of dull and wiry.

will change its degree of curl to match the rest of your head.

- Wave can help you cope with seasonal variations.

You could be a seasonal wave man. During the warm months your hair will probably have more natural curls. It will hold the shape you comb or brush into it better. It probably looks fuller, too. This is because your hair is absorbing water molecules from the humid air, making it softer, fuller, and wavier.

In the coldest months, hair lies flatter, due to lower humidity and the dry heat you live with indoors. This is when you may need the extra boost of a permanent wave to add a lift to your hair.

- Waves can help you cope with aging hair.

Generally, when men age their hair becomes finer with the passing years, although there are exceptions to this rule. If your hair has become finer over time, or if the natural waviness of your hair has departed, a wave can put these qualities back into your hair.

How to Maintain a Wave

Proper maintenance is *vital* to keeping a wave looking good. Since a wave changes the chemical structure of your hair, the hair shafts are permanently weakened and made more porous; they require extra conditioning. Here is how to maintain your wave so that it looks natural and healthy and gives you all the benefits it can:

The First Forty-eight Hours

Your hair needs to rest for at least forty-eight hours after it has been processed. It needs that long to regain its pH balance, a slightly acidic state that is disrupted by processing. So skip shampooing your hair for two days after it is waved.

What to do those first two days? You can rinse your hair with water, but don't shampoo or use creme rinses or conditioners. To style your newly textured locks, use your fingers or a wide-toothed comb. Don't try to get out all the "snags" in the wave. Just neaten your basic shape and save the brushing and blow-drying for a couple of days. (*Tip:* Have your hair waved on a Friday afternoon, and you will be able to style it Sunday night for work on Monday.)

Shampooing

You want to counter the weakening effects of waving by using a mild shampoo. Waves can rob the hair of the oil that smoothes does the scalelike cuticles of hair shafts. Hair without enough oil looks dull and tends to "flyaway," because individual hair shafts cannot lie down flat against each other when their cuticles are so roughed up.

The shampoo you use on waved hair should contain additives that help the shampoo condition as well as clean. These include citric acid, which helps mend cuticle scales; emollients, which act in place of the hair's natural oils and lock in moisture within hair shafts; and protein, which coats and strengthens porous waved hair. Two shampoos—Clinique's Clean Scalp Shampoo in the Skin Supplies for Men line and Pantene for Men's Vitamin Protein Shampoo—are particularly good for waves because they clean gently but condition thoroughly.

Conditioning

Even if your hair didn't need the extra protec-

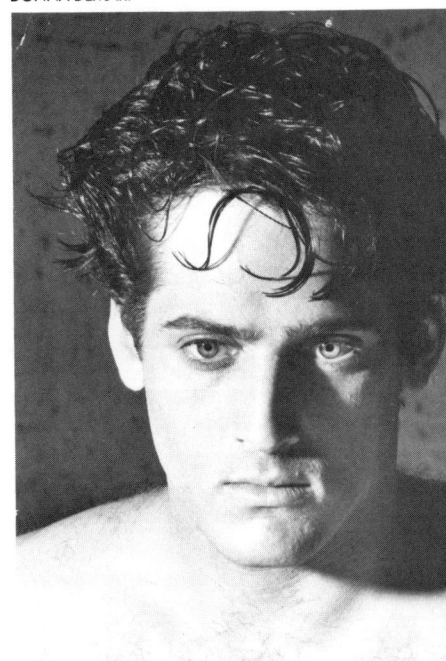

Wavy hair is the most versatile. A simple combing can straighten it entirely or just in sections. With the help of a gel or mousse, the hair can be molded to reflect many different moods—whatever appeals to you at the moment, slick or free-form and left to dry. Wavy hair can be most daring. Play with hair groomers and find your own variation.

tion of an after-shampoo conditioner before it was waved, waved hair needs such care. By coating hair shafts with substances that lock in moisture, coat the hair, fix split ends, and control flyaway strands, conditioners will keep waved hair in top form.

Top performers keeping waved hair problem-free are Aramis's Malt-Enriched Thickening Conditioner, Pantene for Men's Corrector Conditioner, and Redken's Climatress. These add greater manageability, help lessen tangles, control flyaway strands, moisturize, and add lubrication and shine to waved hair.

Regular Hair Cutting Appointments

The problem of split ends is often associated with dry hair. The proper shampoos and conditioners should keep waved hair looking healthy, but once the ends of hair shafts split they can only temporarily be "glued" together by products applied to the hair. Regular trimming (every four to six weeks) will keep split ends from becoming troublesome. Once a week treat your hair to a deep-conditioner, like Redken's Climatress.

There are a multitude of wonders that waves can work for you, and no one will be the wiser. But take your time when deciding whether or not to get a wave. In a way, the process is like plastic surgery. Even if all the changes it brings are favorable, they are still changes you will have to adjust to.

Waves are like plastic surgery in another way: Few procedures can make such a dramatic difference in the way you look. Waves solve hair problems. They can vitalize hair in need of a boost. When your hair is on the line, waves can make the difference between success and mediocrity. That's worth considering.

10.

HAIR COLOR

Subtle New Color Techniques Can Brighten Your Image

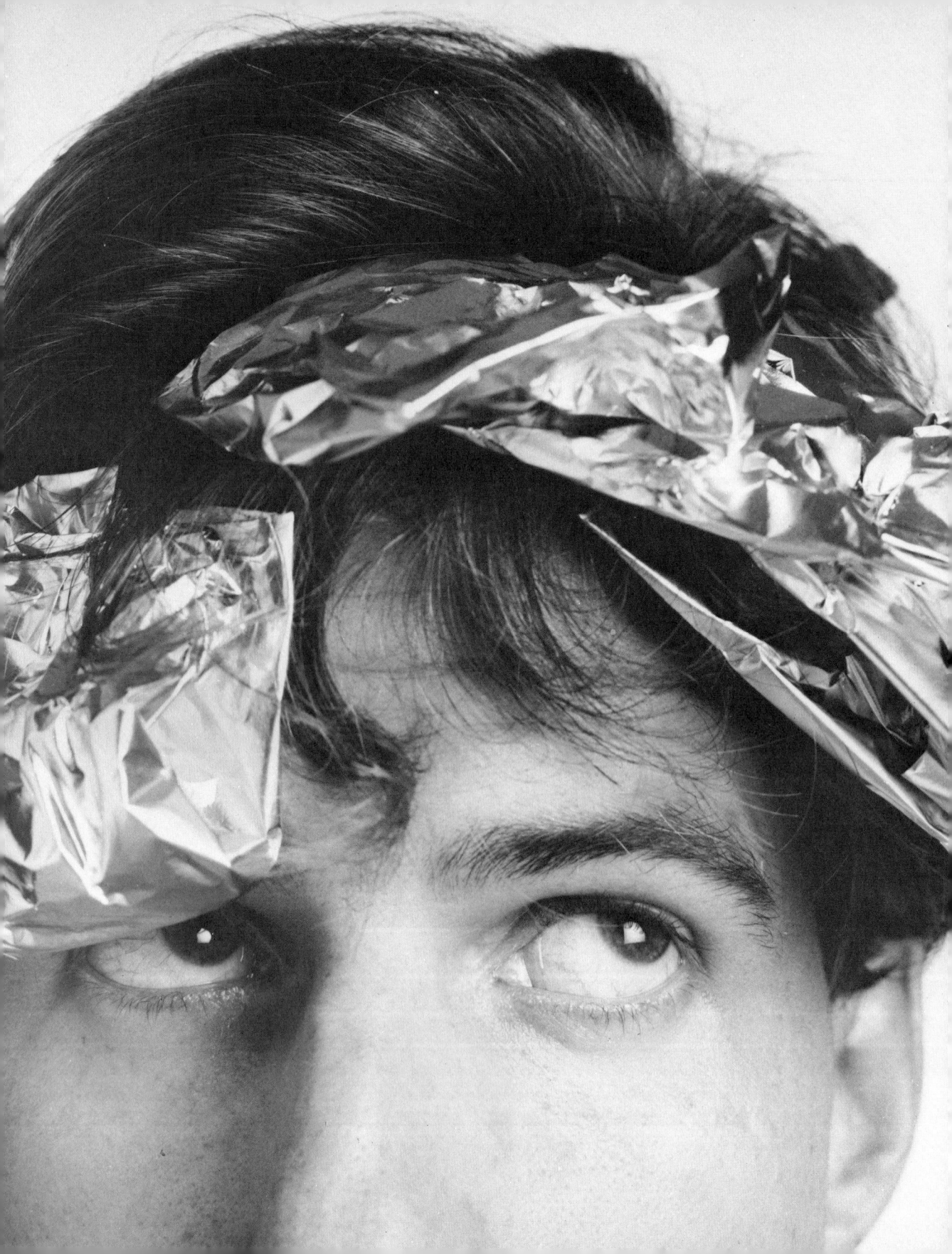

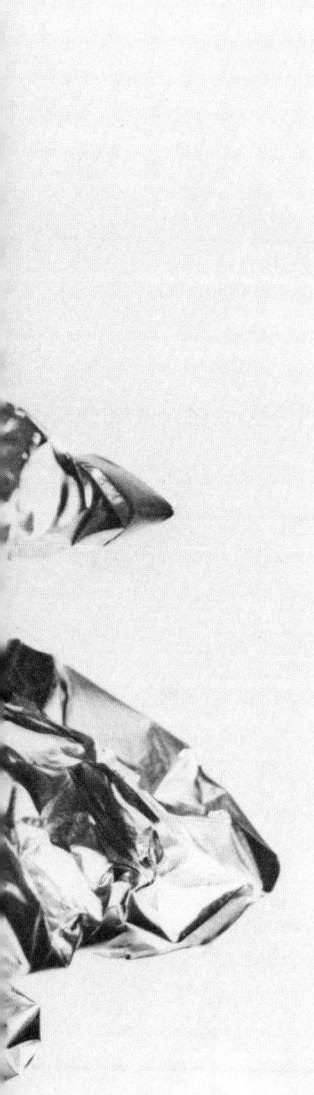

To Color or Not to Color

Somewhere along the line, you will have to make a decision about the color of your hair. The time may come when you start getting gray at the temples and find the effect more aging than flattering and distinguished. It may be when your hair starts thinning and you see too much scalp through the strands. Or it may be when—even though you have a full head of hair in good condition with an excellent cut—you find your hair somehow lacks zip and shine.

Look at the hair of a young child. It's burnished, with a natural, healthy shine. It glows with a depth of color that comes from nature's blend of many subtle shades. That's what to aim for. Your hair stylist can give you realistic color with a glow your hair hasn't had for years.

When you consider the pros and cons of color, forget the artificial obvious dye jobs of the past, those fake shoe polish shades. Hair coloring techniques have changed. Hair coloring is now more *believable* than ever.

Some Color Considerations

The Shine Factor

The key to healthy-looking hair color is shine. There is nothing more aging than flat, dull, unshiny hair. When hair shines, it is vibrant; the color comes alive. Check to see how much shine your hair still has. The best places to look are under the bathroom light or in sunlight. The shinier your hair, the more it will reflect the light. Straight hair tends to be more shiny than curly hair, because it bounces light like a flat piece of glass. Curlier hair will reflect the light less, just as a twisted glass rod will give less reflection.

While you're in a brightly lit place, notice all the colors of your hair that make up its basic shade. You may see variations of light and dark brown, gold, red, white. This blending is what makes your hair look natural. Remember this when you think about coloring your hair.

The Shade Factor

In coloring, you don't ever want a completely solid color. That is what used to make dye jobs so obvious—they didn't allow for any color variation. You've seen that your natural hair is actually a combination of many shades, never just brown, red, or blond. For example, light brown hair usually has many blond strands in it. Blonds may have some brown, gold, white, and red. Dark brown hair usually includes several shades of red in its total color.

Your hair color can also give you the benefit of some optical illusions. Light hair will reflect the light, make your hair and your face look fuller. Lighter hair above the forehead will *lift* the face, make it appear longer. Lighter hair at the temples can visually widen a narrow face, which is why so many men look great with silver sideburns. A lighter hair color can make thinning hair less noticeable by lessening the contrast between hair and scalp.

When many men first think of coloring their hair, they think of returning to the color of their youth. A former New York governor, Hugh Carey, made this mistake, showing up with bright auburn hair that was a radical transformation from his graying locks. His hair color became news and generally got bad reviews, doing nothing for his political image.

Go for a subtle, gradual change rather than an instant transformation. Sometimes going only a few shades lighter can take years off your face. I always advise lighter shades for older clients, to soften any harsh lines in the face.

You should know that hair does not go from light to dark or vice versa instantly with any coloring technique. It must first go through a whole range of shades one by one, before the final color develops.

There is a big difference in the way I color straight or curly hair. The flat surface of straight hair, which reflects more light, will need the most subtle effects. Color can easily look garish or phony, if the wrong shade is chosen.

Curly hair, because it bends the light and because there is so much going on with the curl, can take a more dramatic look, more definite color variations.

The Maintenance Factor

Whenever you consider doing anything that changes your hair, you must consider the upkeep. The key to easy maintenance when coloring your hair is to keep the color changes subtle.

I'll show you subtle color techniques that will give you the healthy youthful look you're after,

The darker the hair, the less light reflection

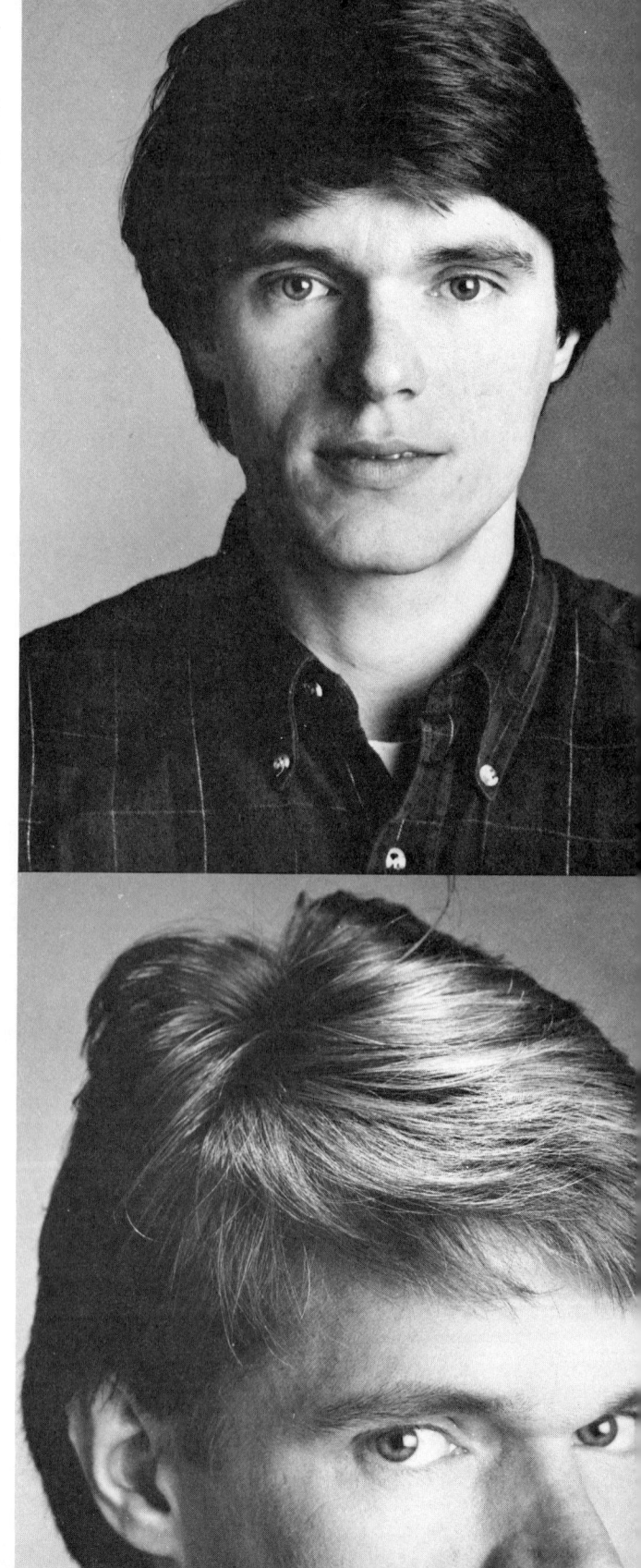

Hair needs light reflection to look shiny and healthy. The darker your hair is, starting from dark blond on to black, the duller and flatter your hair will look. Subtle, lighter colors woven through your hair will make it look fuller and more alive. Don't worry about roots. You won't need a touch-up for at least five months, if ever.

with only a touch-up every four months, if at all.

What Kind of Hair Coloring Is Right for You?

Before you take the plunge into a new hair color, there is a way to preview some of the color effects I'll be talking about. Here's how:

The Color Preview

In most drugstores, you can find a product called a temporary color rinse. I've found that the best available is Fanci-full by Roux. This will coat the hair shafts with a thin film of color pigment. Underneath, the hair remains in its original state.

Use a temporary color rinse to help you see if erasing your silver sideburns or adding red or gold highlights gives your hair the right lift. You won't be able to preview streaking effects or a radical change of color, but you will get an idea of natural, subtle changes.

Temporary color rinses are easy to use. Just dab the liquid on freshly shampooed, damp hair with a cotton ball, straight from the bottle. Work from the roots of the hair to the ends. Then, using a wide toothed comb, blend the color throughout the hair for even distribution.

This technique is messy. Be sure to color your hair at the bathroom sink, in front of a mirror. Go shirtless, to avoid coloring your clothes. Afterwards, dry your hair as usual. If you don't like the results, hop in the shower and in minutes your hair will be back to its original shade.

You may like the effect so much that you are tempted to use this product regularly. If so, there are disadvantages to consider.

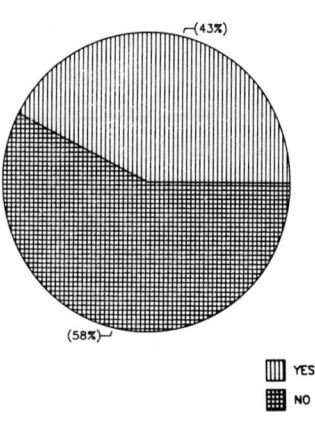

(43%)

(58%)

▦ YES
▦ NO

• The color must be reapplied after every shampoo. It does not penetrate the hair shaft and will wash out in the shower.

• Some temporary color may rub off on your clothing and pillow cases.

• If you are caught in the rain without an umbrella or you're having a strenuous workout at the gym or on the tennis court, you may end up literally dripping with color.

Use temporary color rinses for a special effect, for a preview of more permanent changes to follow, for a one-day-only lift. They're an easy do-it-yourself operation. For more permanent results, using the techniques we'll be discussing from here on, you need a professional's touch.

Who Should Color Your Hair?

Many men enlist their friends, wives, or girl friends to act as at-home colorists. Since most hair coloring products are aimed at women and perhaps the woman in your life colors her own hair successfully, why not let her color yours? You may well reason, especially if she offers with well-meaning enthusiasm.

Here's why *not*: I've seen some disastrous results from Saturday night colorists using over-the-counter preparations. You risk getting a fake-looking flat color or orange, green, or spotty hair. Leaving the mixture on too long can ruin the condition of your hair. Leaving it on for too short a time can give you the wrong color.

Most hair colorists custom-mix their colors, using a formula that is designed especially for you and not available over the counter. They have much experience with timing, which is crucial in hair color, and know just how long to leave the mixture on for the best effect. So leave your hair coloring to the experts, at least the first few times. If you insist on doing it yourself, have a pro teach you how.

Semipermanent Color Washes

These products are applied to the entire head of hair at the same time, coating the hair shafts so they will not rub off on clothes or drip off in the rain. They can give good, rich colors, terrific shine, and more body to the hair.

They will, however, eventually wash out of the hair. Some color is lost with each shampoo, and your hair will return to its natural shade within four to eight shampoos.

If you have light hair and use a blond wash, your hair will acquire a golden shine. Darker hair that is treated with chocolate brown wash will have a new, subtle warmth.

As semipermanent color washes are very tricky to apply, you should *have a hair stylist do it for you or show you how.* The liquid is very messy and can stain the skin if it drips off the hair, creating some hard-to-explain spots on your face. You must also be sure to have the right color for your hair, because the preparation will *not* shampoo out immediately.

Yes, I know there are many hair coloring products that are advertised as "easy to do at home." Don't believe them. It takes coordination and timing to do hair coloring right. So don't cut costs here. No man can afford phony-looking hair color. Find a stylist who specializes in hair color and let him or her do it at least the first few times. I know I

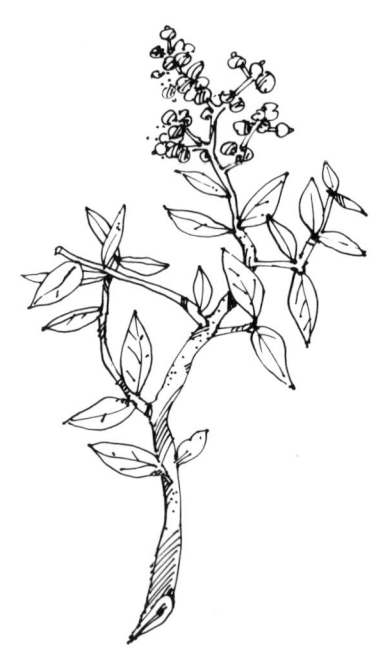

warned you about this before, but it bears repeating.

Henna

Henna is another semipermanent hair coloring. The difference is that henna is a completely natural vegetable dye, derived from the leaves of a shrub growing in parts of Africa and the Near East. It's not only an organic hair colorer, but a natural conditioner, too.

Henna will add body to your hair by coating the hair shafts, bulking them up. And it adds a terrific shine by filling in the cracks in your hair shafts' cuticles, creating a smooth, light-reflecting surface.

Henna comes only in three shades: black, red, and neutral. The neutral type is particularly useful, because it adds body, condition, and shine to hair without changing its color.

Although many henna products are sold for home use, I recommend they be applied only three to four times a year by a professional. He or she will mix the henna powder with hot water and perhaps add some herbs and spices to form a paste, then paint this mixture on your damp hair. After the color or shine has set for a certain length of time (the longer it's on, the deeper the color), he or she will shampoo the mixture out.

As with man-made coloring products, henna must be used correctly for the best results. In fact, in this case, Mother Nature is more powerful than many man-made colorings. The colored henna products must be *carefully timed,* or the color will turn out too strong, with a harsh orange-red hue rather than a burnished glow. Henna can also build up on the strands and throw off the color and texture of the hair.

Lightening Techniques

Natural-looking highlights—making it appear that you've spent time at the beach—are easy to achieve. They don't dramatically alter your hair, and they give the kind of athletic, healthy look many men are after these days.

Here's an easy trick you can do yourself. If you are planning to be out in the sun, make the sun work to create highlights for you. Comb straight lemon juice (for stronger highlights) or a water/lemon juice mixture (for softer streaks) through your hair before hitting the beach. The lemon juice will lighten your hair naturally, without giving you the peroxided surfer look of the '60s.

I give my clients who are not playing in the sun the healthy look of someone who is by one of two techniques. I lighten the hair at the top, sides, and front by applying a lighter shade of single-process permanent coloring (discussed below) with my fingers, to be sure the placement of color is natural. After the coloring is processed, I give them a shampoo.

The second technique is almost like painting color in the hair. It's called *foil highlighting*. Small sections of hair from around your head are combed out and painted with a brush. The painted sections are then wrapped in foil while they process.

I might use several different shades on each head of hair—bronze tints on brown hair, white or gold on blonds. After a shampoo your hair will have highlights framing your face, but the look will be natural because its placement has been controlled.

DONNA DEMARI

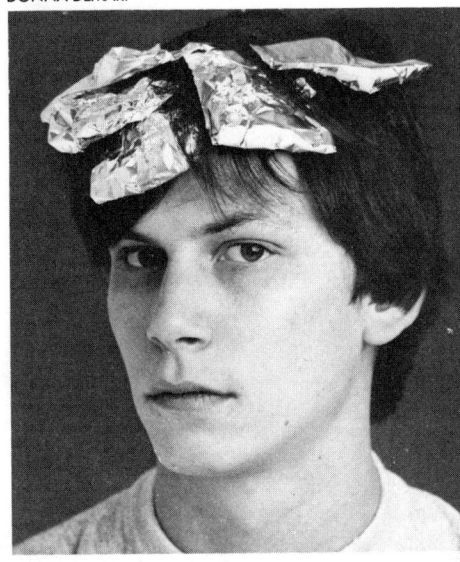

Remember the word dye? That was in the '50s. Today's hair color looks believable and natural—you look like you've been sailing in the Caribbean for a month. Brighten your overall image with the subtlest amount of warmth added to your hair and you can also mask the gray. Here you see one method of brightening the hair: foil highlighting.

223

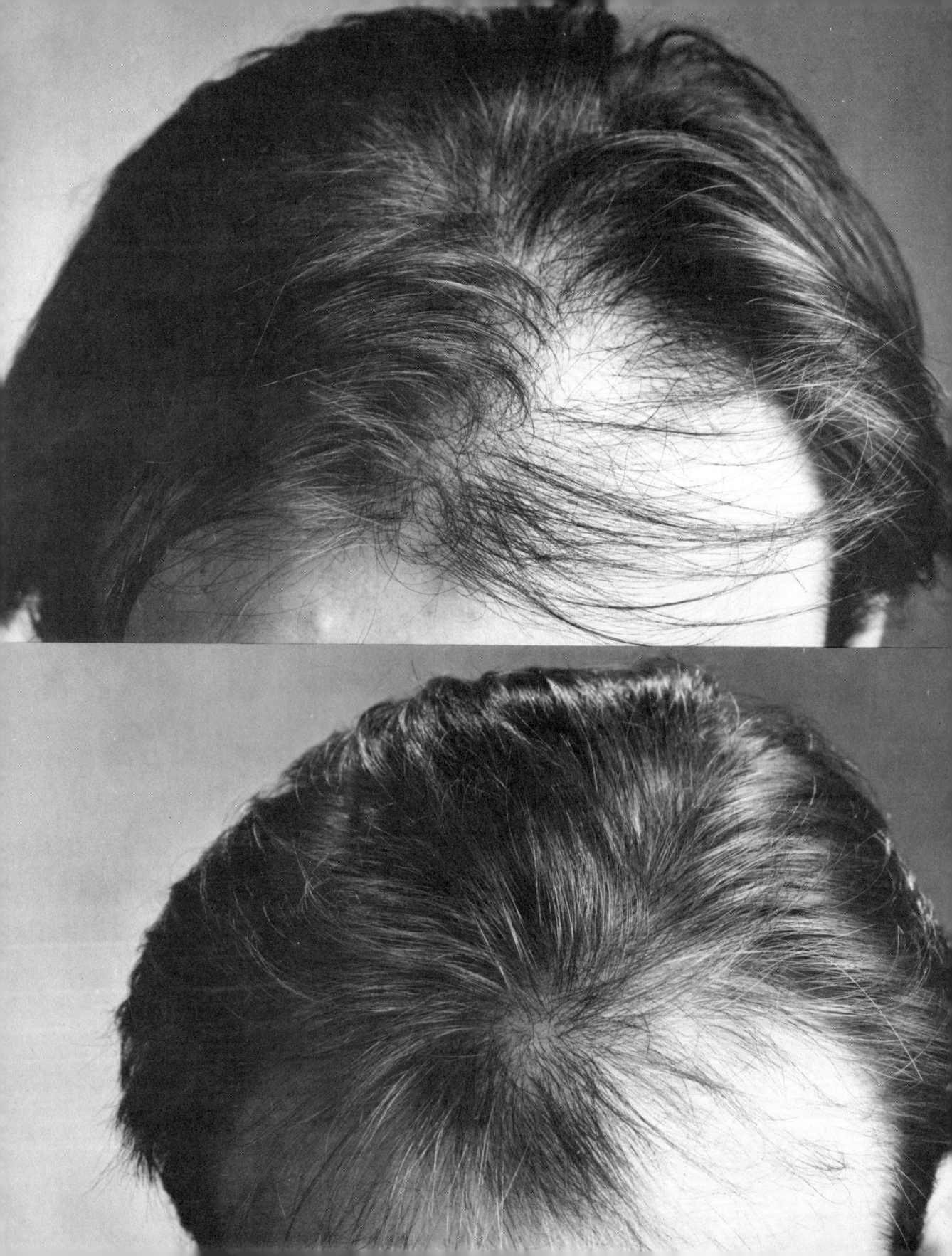

Highlights and Hairlines

Another use of highlights is to help men camouflage receding hairlines. If there is too much contrast between the balding area and the scalp, your hair will look even more sparse. Highlighting this area with a lighter color will lessen the contrast, making hair appear fuller and thicker.

I used this technique on a well-known Manhattan dentist, Dr. Richard Crystal. I lightened the medium-brown base color of his hair to a subtle light brown and then added red blond highlights to the thinning area. It looks as if he had spent a sunny weekend sailing. Now he wears his hair a bit shorter. It looks much thicker, with less contrast between hair and scalp.

Single-Process Permanent Coloring

In order to permanently recolor hair, a coloring solution must penetrate hair shafts, altering the pigment contained *within* rather than just coating the surface. The hair remains processed until new hair grows out.

You can use single-process hair coloring instead of temporary color washes because you want to *keep* your new hair color. The peroxide in these products will oxidize your hair's natural color, while the coloring solution penetrates hair shafts and recolors the pigment granules there in a single step. Single-process permanent coloring can lighten (or darken) your hair by several shades on the color scale. It will not create a drastic change, such as from lightest blond to darkest brown or vice versa.

If you are interested in any permanent coloring technique, your stylist should perform a strand test on a sample of your hair. This will give the colorist all the information needed to judge what colors to use and how long to leave them on your hair. But be warned: Once your hair is permanently colored, your maintenance time escalates. New color will have to be applied to your hair's roots every four to seven weeks.

Double-Process Permanent Coloring

The most radical (and therefore least advisable by far) coloring technique is really only practical for dark-haired men who want to become completely blond. Frankly, I never recommend it. The results are usually phony-looking, and it tends to ruin the texture and condition of the hair.

In the first step of double processing, called the

bleach out, a lightener/peroxide solution strips hair of its color. Once prelighted, a coloring agent called a *toner* colors the prelighted hair to the desired blond shade.

Double-process hair coloring really beats up on hair, and the maintenance to keep such hair in proper condition is time-consuming. If you insist on this despite my warning, find the best colorist in town and let him or her handle the procedure.

Covering Your Gray Hair

I wanted to give the subject of gray hair its own section in this book because it's one of the main reasons men color their hair.

Unfortunately, many men pick the absolute worst method for ridding themselves of gray. I'm talking about those "just comb through your hair" products often advertised on television.

Men are lead to believe these lotions restore hair color naturally. Forget it. These solutions are lead compounds dissolved in water and alcohol. They coat hair with a dull film of metallic salt. All natural highlights and shading tones are covered. Result: Hair shaft cuticles are coated with a slick, oily, fake-looking sludge. Don't do it!

There are much better ways to cover gray. A temporary color wash about two shades lighter than your natural hair color (still much darker than your gray hair) will hide the gray subtly and preview a more permanent coloring technique. Just dab the solution directly on the gray area with cotton balls. But remember, this color will wash out with shampoos, showers, rain, and sweat, so use it as a preview—or to cover gray just for the day.

Your best bet for long-term results is to use a semipermanent color wash one or two shades lighter than your natural hair color. This will soften the overall look of your hair while covering the gray with a light tone. And because the gray in your hair will be lighter than the rest of your hair, (remember, semipermanent colors only slightly penetrate hair shafts, so variations in color will occur in the hair) you will get great-looking highlights.

This method of covering gray is sure to avoid the "dye job" look. The perfect time to use semipermanent color on your gray is during a vacation. You leave pale and gray, return to work suntanned and much younger-looking.

Toners for Great-Looking Gray

Many men with gray or white hair quite rightly enjoy their hair's basic color but don't like the yellowish cast it often develops.

There are several reasons your hair may have yellowed. One is a matter of the hair's natural pigment. Or it could be a buildup on the hair shaft of pollutants such as cigarette smoke. Or there could be a buildup of hair products: shampoo residue, conditioners, hair groomers, and sprays.

To strip this buildup from your gray hair, you can use something you may already have in your house: lemon juice or vinegar. After shampooing, rinse your hair with a fifty-fifty solution of lemon juice (or vinegar) and water. Do this once a day for four days. It should remove any environmental buildup on the hair.

If the acid rinses of lemon juice or vinegar don't work, then chances are your discoloration is caused by the pigments within the hair shaft. In this case, look for a gray toner on your drugstore shelves. Pick a silver or white color and apply this to freshly shampooed hair. Or better yet, have a professional colorist do it for you—you'll be sure to get the right shade. These toners contain no peroxide, so there will be no change in the structure of your hair. You'll leave them on from five to twenty minutes, according to the package directions. Rinse, and say good-bye to yellow.

Darkening Your Eyebrows

If your eyebrows are too light from being exposed to the sun or you feel that darker brows would add to your face, here's an easy technique to darken them subtly.

Take a light brown or charcoal gray eyebrow pencil and wet it. Then rub the pencil on the bristles of an old toothbrush so the color comes off on the bristles. Then lightly brush your brows upward. Just enough of the pencil color should get on the brows for a very discreet darkening of color.

Some Final Thoughts on Coloring

Great-looking, believable, vibrant hair color can be yours easily.

So consider the potential of today's new hair coloring products to give your hair youthful shine and bounce, to give you natural highlighting effects that will play up your best features, "zip up" your skin tone, improve your whole appearance.

It could be just what your hair needs. In any case, it's a great option for *every* man to consider.

11

SKIN CARE

Skin Care Is Simple and Direct . . . and It Really Works

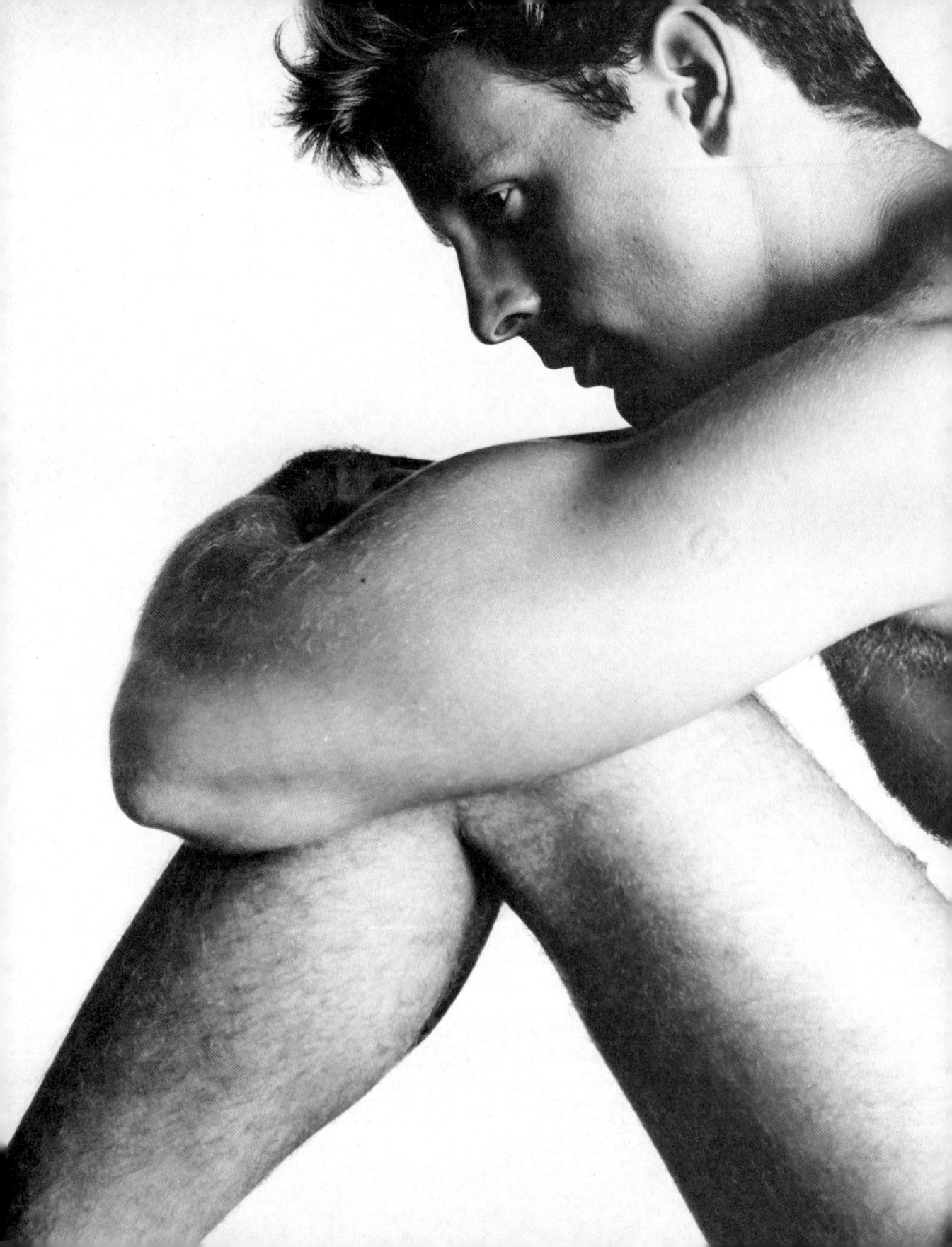

Your Skin Care Strategy

Everyone is born with great-looking skin, but from childhood on, your skin is threatened by pollution, poor diet, sun exposure, tension, medication, and central heating. All of this happens in addition to the natural aging process.

It's easy to take for granted all the wonderful things your skin does. It is the largest organ of your body and works hard to protect you against chemical and bacterial invasions. It's a shock absorber for your internal organs; it stores fats, water, and minerals; it rids your body of toxic wastes; it's a great sensory organ; it has the capacity to repair and restore itself; it is totally waterproof.

You owe it to your health to care for your skin as much as you owe it to your looks. Your skin is one of the first places to show any kind of illness or internal distress. It's also quick to show signs of neglect. I've discovered how you can have great-looking skin. It's not complicated. You won't have to spend a lot of money. Skin care is simple and direct, and it really works.

As with your hair, the condition of your skin can range from dry to oily, with normal skin lying somewhere in between. Some men's faces are dry on the cheeks and oily on the nose, chin, and forehead. Before deciding which products to use, you should determine your skin type. Here are some guidelines:

Normal to Dry Skin

- You have small pores and little surface moisture.
- Your skin has a flat, nonshiny surface.
- You may have lines and wrinkles at an early age.
- You may have skin irritations due to razor drag.
- You have trouble getting a close shave.
- Your skin sometimes feels tight and constricted after washing.

Normal to Oily Skin

- You have large pores.
- Your face—especially the nose, chin, and forehead—gets surface moisture and oil.
- You occasionally have blackheads, whiteheads, and blemishes.
- Your face often looks shiny.

Combination Skin

- You have both dry and oily skin characteristics.
- Your skin looks oily on the T zone across the forehead and down the nose to the chin.
- Your cheeks can be dry and flaky, and your undereye area can be dry and prone to wrinkles.

Note: All skin types can vary with season, climate, age, stress, hormonal changes, diet, or health. Your skin is like a barometer telling what's going on in the rest of your body.

Caring for your skin need not be a complicated routine. Basically all you need do is follow three simple steps: cleansing, toning, and moisturizing. Whenever you think of cleaning your face, think

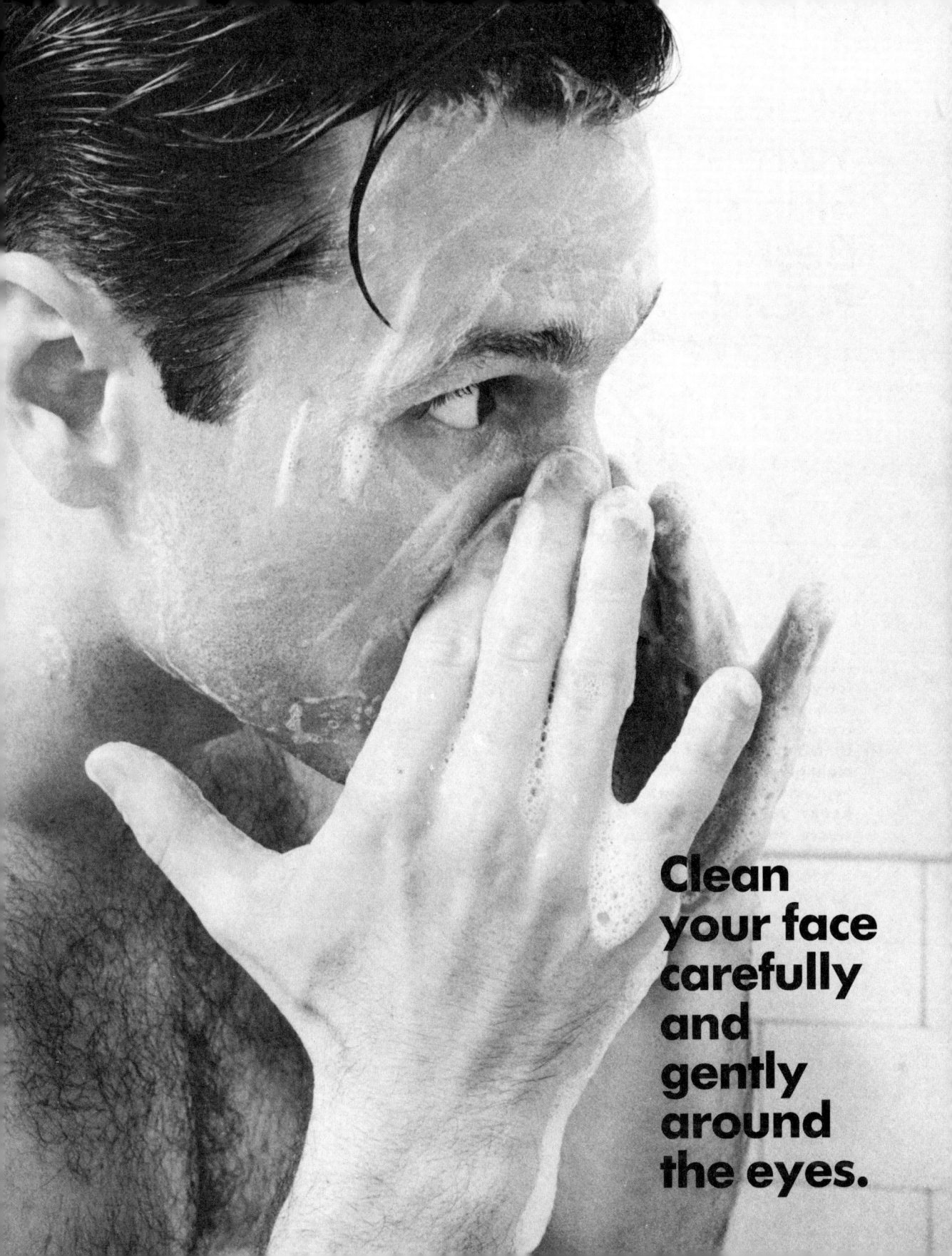

Clean your face carefully and gently around the eyes.

Water,
Your
Skin's
Best
Friend

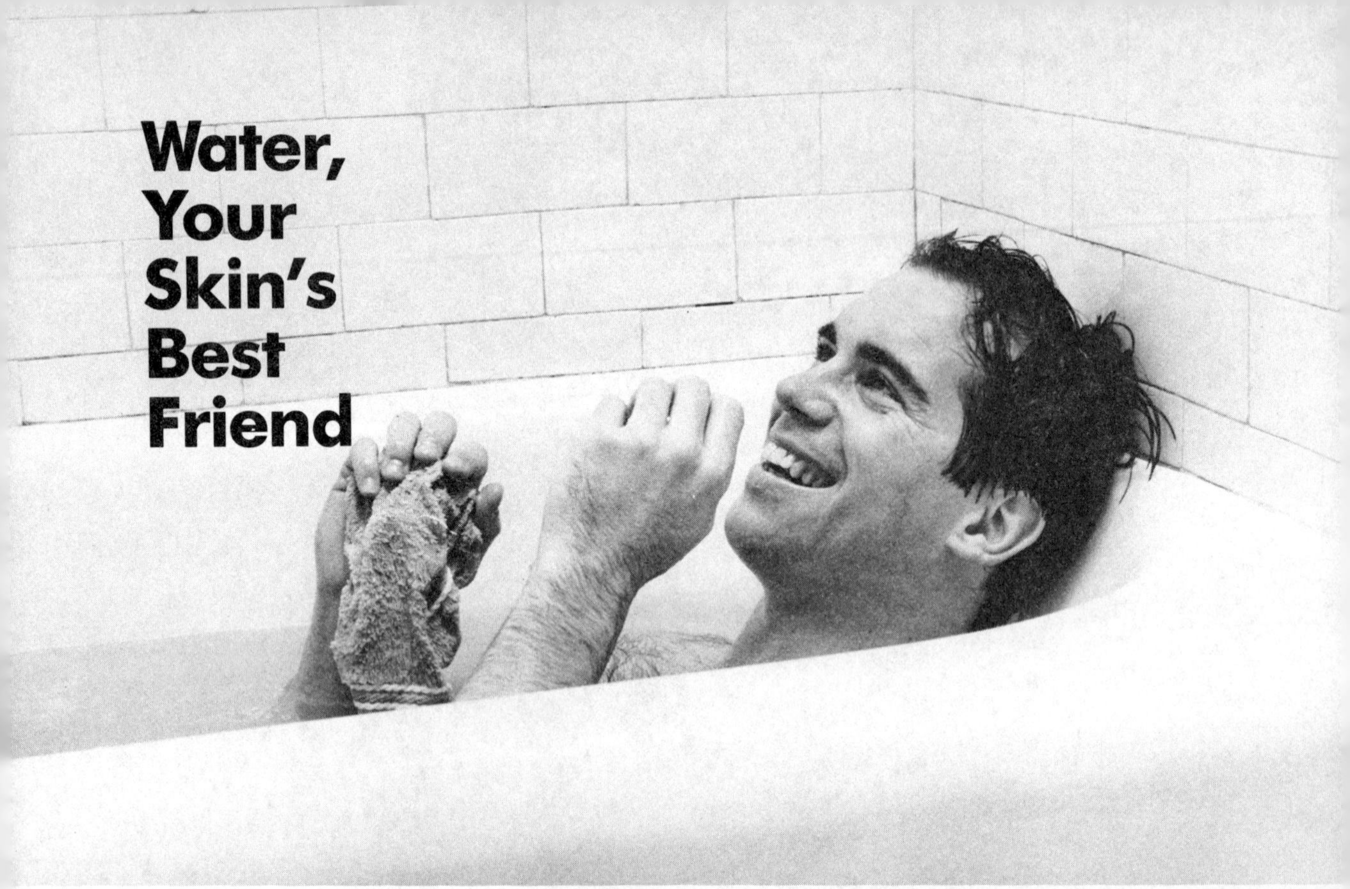

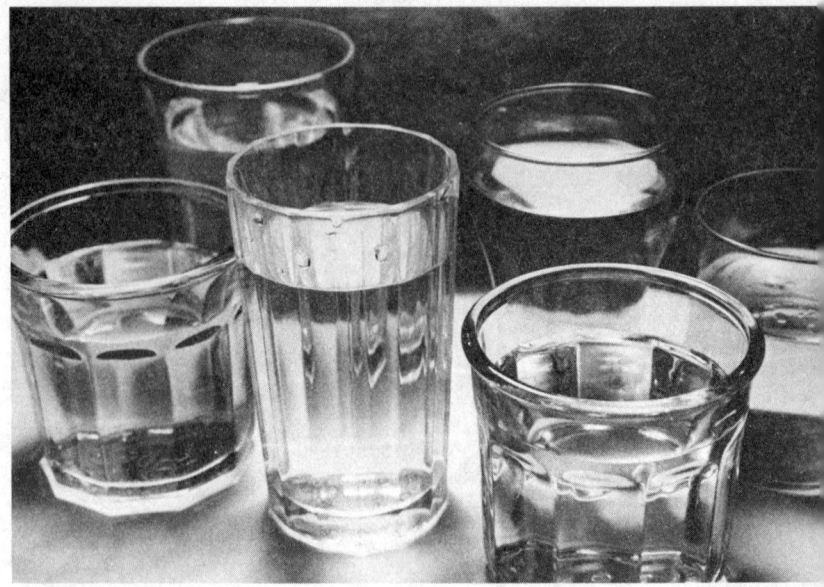

The best thing you can do for your skin is to supply it with water, both internally and externally. Drinking lots of water—at least six to eight glasses a day—flushes impurities from the system, keeps your sweat glands clean, and supplies your skin with moisture from the inside. From the outside, do all you can to get moisture into your skin, especially if it is dry. Clean and rinse your face thoroughly. Use moisturizer after shaving. If the air in your home is dry, treat yourself to a humidifier and keep it going in the bedroom at night.

RANDY DUNBAR

234

of these three steps. Make them automatic, as much a part of your life as brushing your teeth.

Skin Care Basics: Cleansing

You skin builds up a sludge composed of sweat, oil, environmental pollutants, and dead skin cells, all of which can make it look thick and coarse. If this sludge isn't flushed away, the pores become clogged and cause blemishes.

Soap and nonsoap cleansers perform two essential functions at the same time. They mix with oil, grease, and other waste substances lying around on your skin and lift them from the surface so that, when you rinse your face, a thin layer of dead skin cells and any dirt, sweat, sebum, and bacteria lying on your skin is picked up and carried away.

Cleansing Normal Skin

I suggest using a nonsoap cleansing bar instead of soap. (A good one is made by Pierre Cattier for Nature de France—available at health food stores.) This will leave less residue on the surface of your skin than most soaps. Soap leaves a film, and you need many rinses to remove the residue.

Lather your face in a circular upward motion. Then rinse your face thoroughly with warm water.

Cleansing Oily Skin

Using the same method as for normal skin, you may substitute a mild transparent glycerin bar such as Pears Soap or Neutrogena. To help break up the oils and prevent spots and blackheads from forming, you may use a complexion brush or loofah with your cleanser. This really gets into the pores to clean them. Use a *gentle* circular motion. Hard scrubbing overstimulates the oil glands, producing more outbreaks. Easy does it.

DO YOU MOISTURIZE YOUR SKIN?

(49%)

(51%)

▥ YES
▦ NO

Cleansing Dry Skin

Dry skin must be given the gentlest care possible. You must choose your cleanser carefully to guard against ingredients that might irritate your skin or dry it more. I suggest a nonsoap cleansing bar made by Rainbow, available at health food stores; a super-fatted soap such as Basis Soap; or an olive oil soap such as Kiss My Face, also available at health food stores. Look for nonperfumed soaps, because perfumes can irritate some skins. Use the same washing procedure described under normal skin, being sure to rinse thoroughly (splash ten to twenty times).

Cleansing Combination Skin

Use the same method as cleansing oily skin.

Skin Care Basics: Toning

Toning your skin stimulates and tightens the pores after the skin has been properly cleansed, and it prepares the skin for the moisturizer. It also removes the final residue of cleanser. If you have dry, normal, or combination skin, use a toner that has no alcohol. The only skin type that should use a toner with alcohol is oily skin. The procedure: Simply soak a cotton ball with your toner and wipe your face until the cotton ball comes away clean.

Skin Care Basics: Moisturizing

A major consideration in skin care is keeping skin moist. Dry skin can look gray, flaky, and rough because dead skin cells lie compressed on the surface of the skin like balloons without air. Once plumped with water, they give a smoother, more even appearance. Moisturizer applied over your

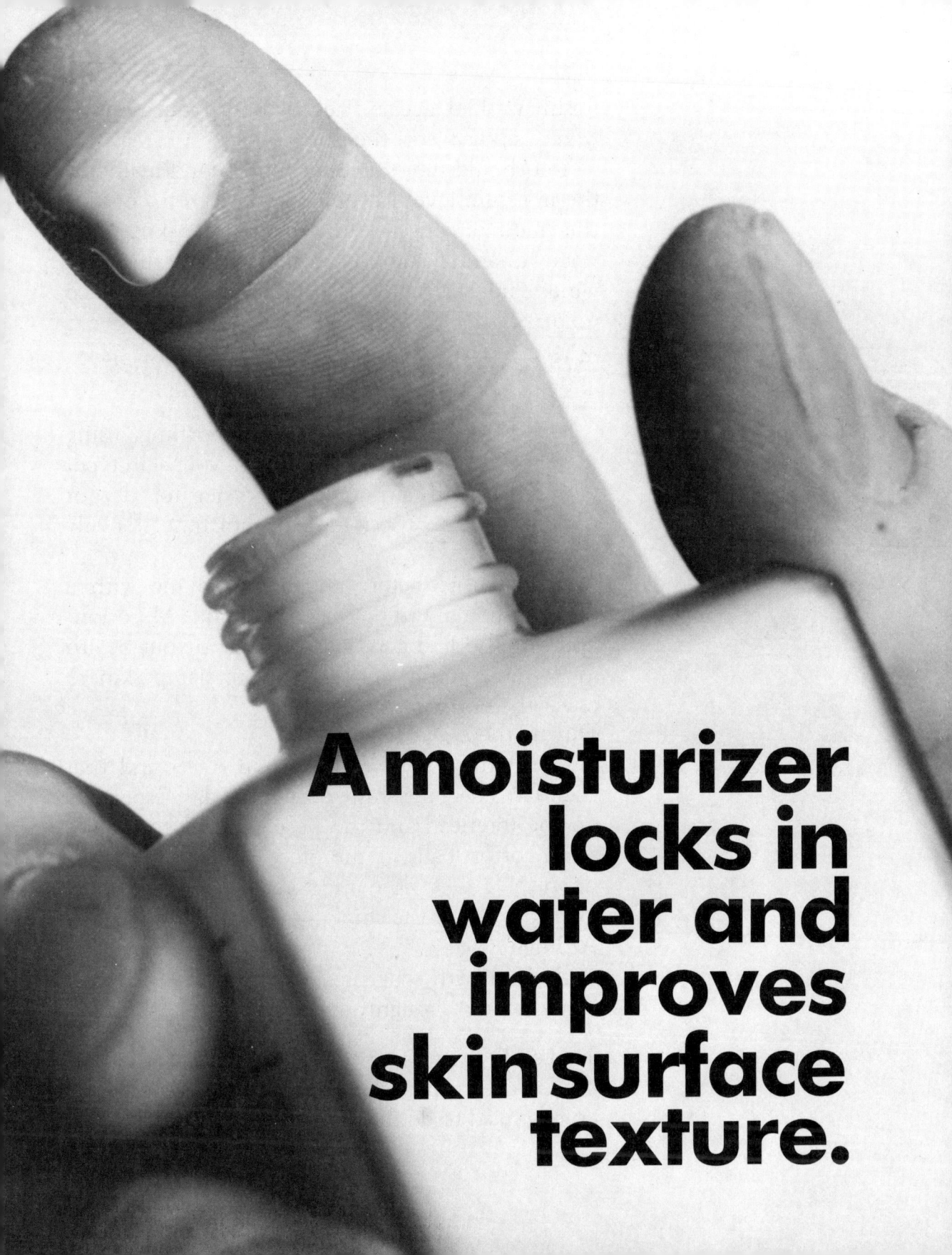

A moisturizer locks in water and improves skin surface texture.

freshly washed face and neck works to trap as much water as possible in the skin.

You should moisturize to nourish and maintain the moisture level in the upper layers of the skin; the moisturizer should leave your skin soft, smooth, and flexible. It will combat attacks of wind, cold, sun, and aging and improve the surface texture of the skin.

An Easy Routine for All Skin Types

A.M. Wakeup

- Wash before shaving in the morning, using soap or a cleansing bar according to your skin type.
- Tone with a nonalcohol toner for dry or normal skin, an (optional) alcohol toner for oily skin.
- Moisturize before and after shaving with a product such as Oil of Olay or Clinique M Lotion. You can also find good moisturizers in your health food store. Apply enough to your damp skin to cover the entire face.

During the Day

Men with overactive oily skin often find that their faces become shiny during the day, especially on the forehead and the nose. Keep a toner and some cotton balls at the office and, in the afternoon, give your nose and forehead a quick once-over to wipe off the shine.

At Night

Cleanse with soap or a nonsoap cleansing bar. Rinse extra thoroughly and moisturize.

That's all there is to it. Taking care of the skin basics—cleansing, toning, moisturizing—is all you usually need to do to keep your skin good-looking.

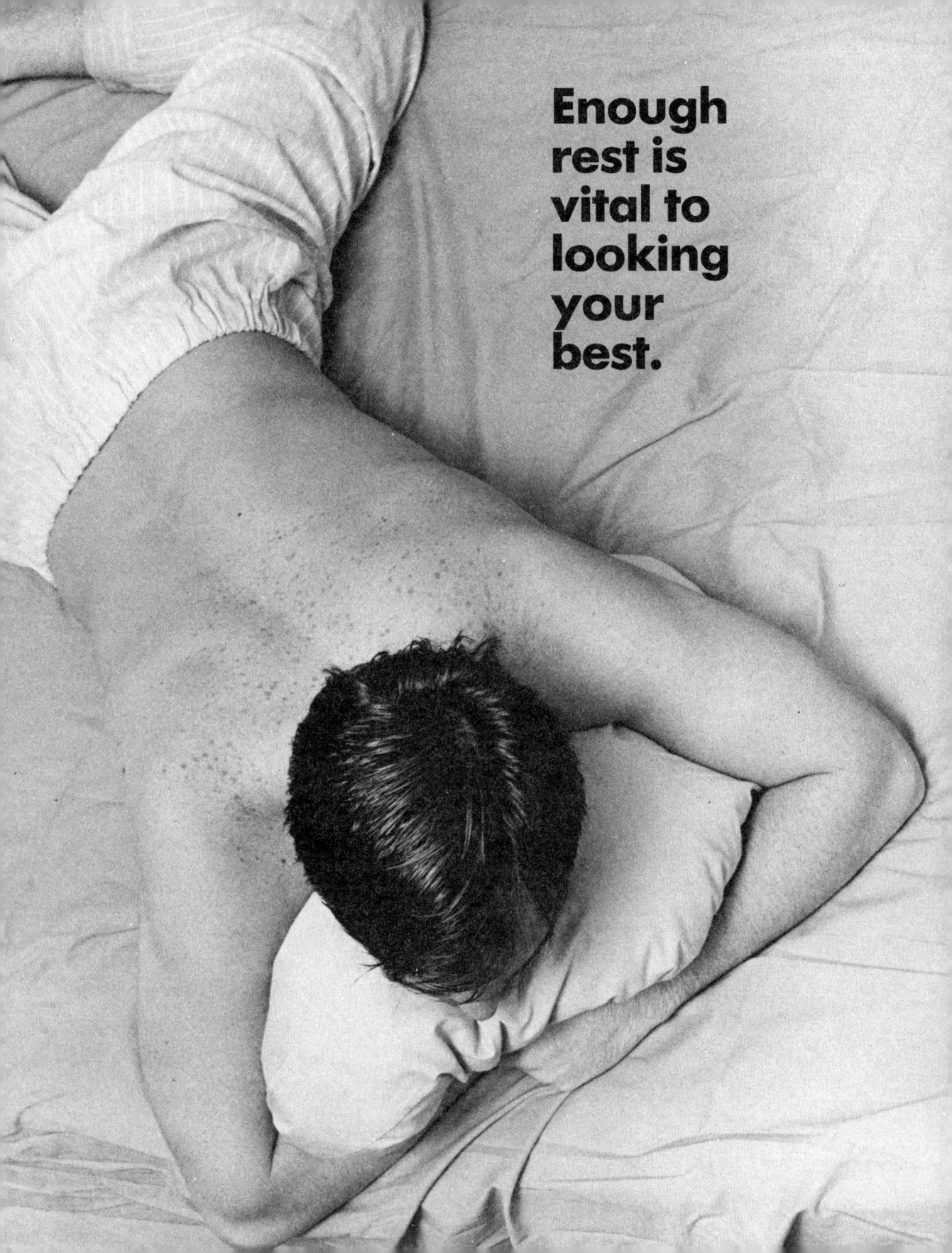

Enough rest is vital to looking your best.

Special Skin Care Products

Once in a while, your skin may need extra help. This happens if you have had exposure to harsh weather conditions or if a buildup of debris on the surface of your skin is clogging the pores. Then you may want to explore some other skin care products that have proven helpful in improving skin conditions.

Facial Scrubs

Facial scrubs consist of tiny grains that are suspended in a semiliquid base. Most contain a good scent and a skin refresher such as menthol to give your skin a super clean feeling.

Use a scrub once a week, twice at most. Simply scoop out some of the scrub onto your fingers and rub it into your damp skin with a gentle circular motion. Rinse thoroughly. Then apply moisturizer.

The idea behind facial scrubs is simple. If you can cut through the outer layer of dead skin cells on your face, you will find better skin underneath just waiting to be exposed. Scrubbing your skin unclogs its pores, gives it a new vitality by making it smoother and more translucent. It can actually take on a much healthier glow.

Facial scrubs are often particularly good for older men. Their skin tends to build up more surface cells, which make the skin look leathery. This can be counteracted by removing a top layer of skin.

Once you have removed the top layer of dead skin, the skin underneath is very vulnerable. Protect it by first tightening the pores with a splash of cold water. Then, after patting the face dry, apply a moisturizer.

You should scrub your skin only once or twice a

week and discontinue use if your skin becomes overly sensitive. Clinique for Men makes a good facial scrub.

Facial Masks

Like scrubs, masks remove a layer of dead skin cells. They reach down into pores and extract clogged oil. They stimulate blood circulation. After a mask, your skin will look smoother, fresher, less wrinkled. While all these benefits are only temporary, they can last for several days with regular use.

Tip: To maximize the benefits of a mask, lie down after putting it on and prop your feet up about a foot off the bed or couch. This increases the blood circulation to the face and helps you relax and enjoy the tingling sensation of the mask as it dries.

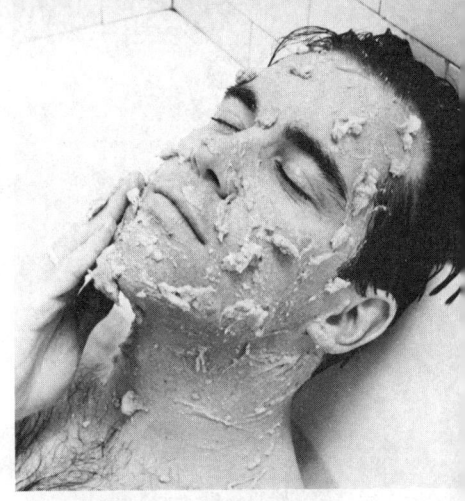

Ever heard of a facial mask? They're available at health food stores and skin salons all over the country. Some are made for use at home, and here's what they will do for you. They clean your pores, remove dead skin cell particles, hydrate your face, and can temporarily tighten the skin. A monthly mask should be part of your skin maintenance routine.

Exercise to Keep Your Skin in Shape

Your body's general fitness and health is reflected in your skin. I've noticed that the men who exercise most seem to have the healthiest skin. It's no mystery why. Exercise makes you perspire, helping to flush your skin of impurities. At the same time, exercise steps up your blood circulation, and improved circulation helps skin stay fit.

Sex and Your Skin

Sex, a wonderful tonic for whatever ails you, is also a real booster for your skin. The benefits derive from two sources: the exercise involved and, more importantly, the orgasmic rush of blood throughout your system, which brings a glow to your skin.

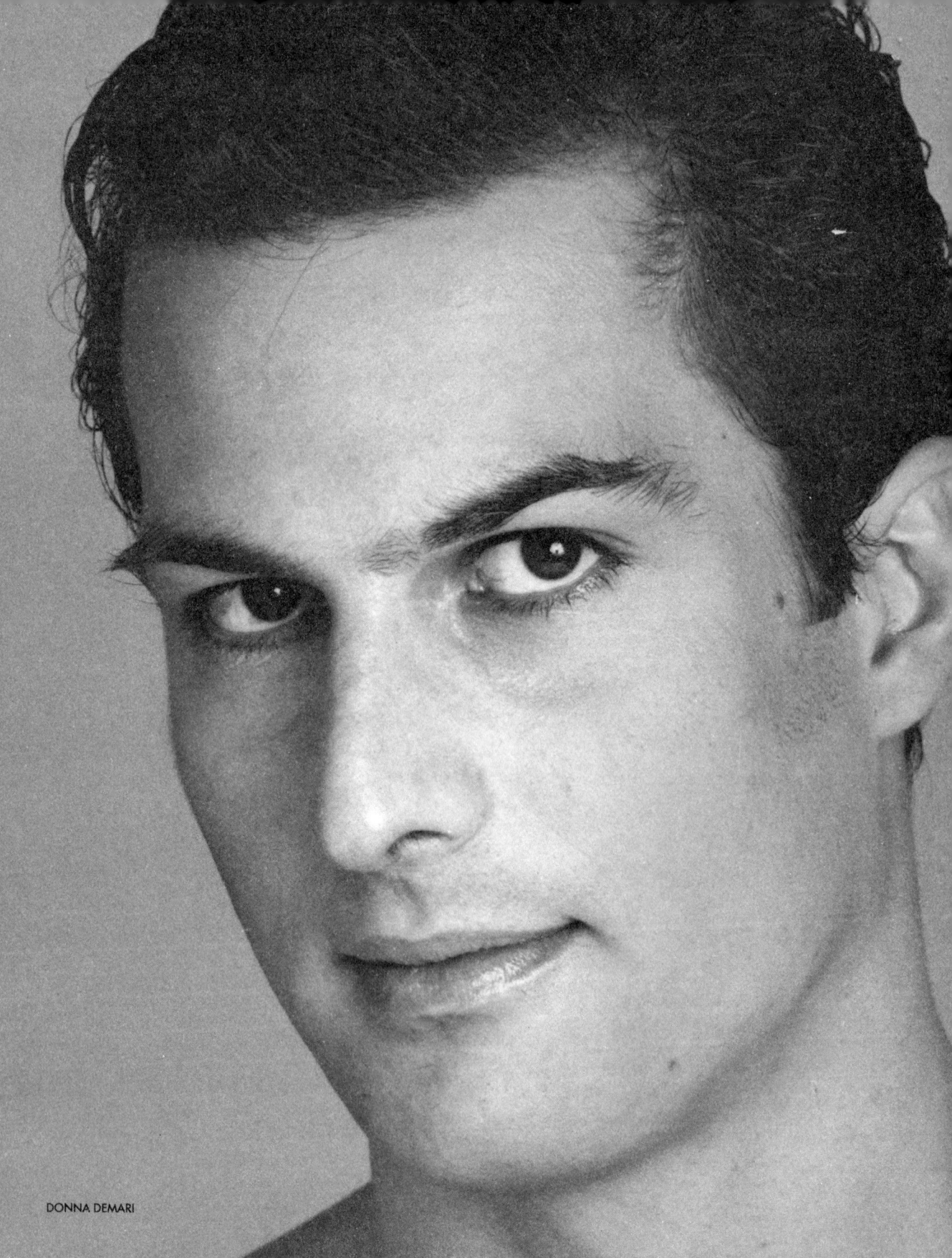

DONNA DEMARI

Keeping Your Skin Calm

Your skin reacts negatively to tension and stress. The most obvious effect is increased oil production, which can trigger acne flare-ups. Today there are enough easy-to-learn relaxation techniques to help you cope with most of stress's bad effects.

Learn to relax. Your skin will reflect your inner calm by becoming tranquil itself.

Protecting Your Skin from the Elements

During very hot or very cold weather, your skin may need extra help. Your skin can cope with changes in climate with a few precautions on your part.

Coping with Cold Weather

During winter months, your body's metabolism slows, reducing the amount of oil produced and constricting the pores carrying this oil to the skin's surface. This double assault can cause your skin to get so dry, flaky, or beaten by the cold that is seems burned.

You can fight chapped skin by helping your skin keep the moisture it has. Use a moisturizer containing more oil to seal and protect the skin.

If you ski, be sure to wear a sun block over your normal moisturizer to counteract the sun's rays, which are quite strong at high altitudes.

Coping with Hot Weather

Exposure to the sun can trigger an increase in oil production and also cause your skin cells to reproduce and shed more quickly. If you suffer from acne, you may find your skin actually becoming drier. Although more oil is produced, the sun also dries the skin, which is good news for acne sufferers.

Your skin is generally dirtier in the summer than at other times of the year. More oil and more sweat lie on top of it, attracting more grit from the environment. You still shouldn't have to wash more than twice a day. However, men with oily skin—and men whose skin is usually normal but has turned oily with the heat—may need to use a toner during the day to take the shine off their faces.

While you might think moisturizers could be put away until fall, you still need them in summer to seal water into the skin. Use the lightest moisturizer possible in the hot months; try one formulated with water as the main ingredient. Its lighter formula should be just right.

The Sun

In recent years, there has been an avalanche of evidence that the sun is definitely harmful to the good health of your skin. Skin cancer due to overexposure to the sun is the greatest potential harm, but any sun at all acts to age the skin prematurely.

Since you probably won't want to sacrifice your tan, you just have to be extra careful. At the beginning of the sunning season, keep your exposure to the sun short—no more than fifteen minutes your first day out, twenty the second, then *gradually* building.

You should never burn your skin. So if you are going to be in the sun for any length of time, use a sun block. Ranging in strength on a scale from 2 to 15 (which blocks all burning rays from your skin), sun blocks are the answer to playing in the sun without paying with the health of your skin. Use them.

Some Very Quiet Helpers

Sometimes your face needs some outside help to look its very best. Anything associated with makeup gives most men the shakes—they say it is unnatural and fake. But some of our most famous politicians and public figures take full advantage of the products on the market that can make a man look healthier, younger, and less tired. So should you when your skin needs to make its best public appearance.

Bronzers

With all the bad press that natural sun tans have received lately, the popularity of bronzers is growing fast. Bronzers give you the look of a great tan without the skin damage of the real thing. Bronzers are harmless transparent gel colorings that will not hide skin imperfections; they just make your skin a few shades darker.

The most common type of bronzer comes in a tube and looks like a gel toothpaste. Aramis, Clinique, and Calvin Klein make good bronzers.

To use a bronzer:

- Stand in front of the bathroom mirror or in front of the mirror in your home with the best light. You'll get the best result by applying bronzer to a freshly washed, shaved, and moisturized face.

- Squeeze a bit of bronzer onto the fingertips of one hand, rub the gel between the fingers of both hands, and spread it across your entire face. It may take a little practice to get the color even. To help even it out, you can mix the bronzer in your hand with a bit of water or moisturizer before applying it to your face. The thinner consistency often blends better.

- Take special care to blend the bronzer into the hairline and the sideburns.

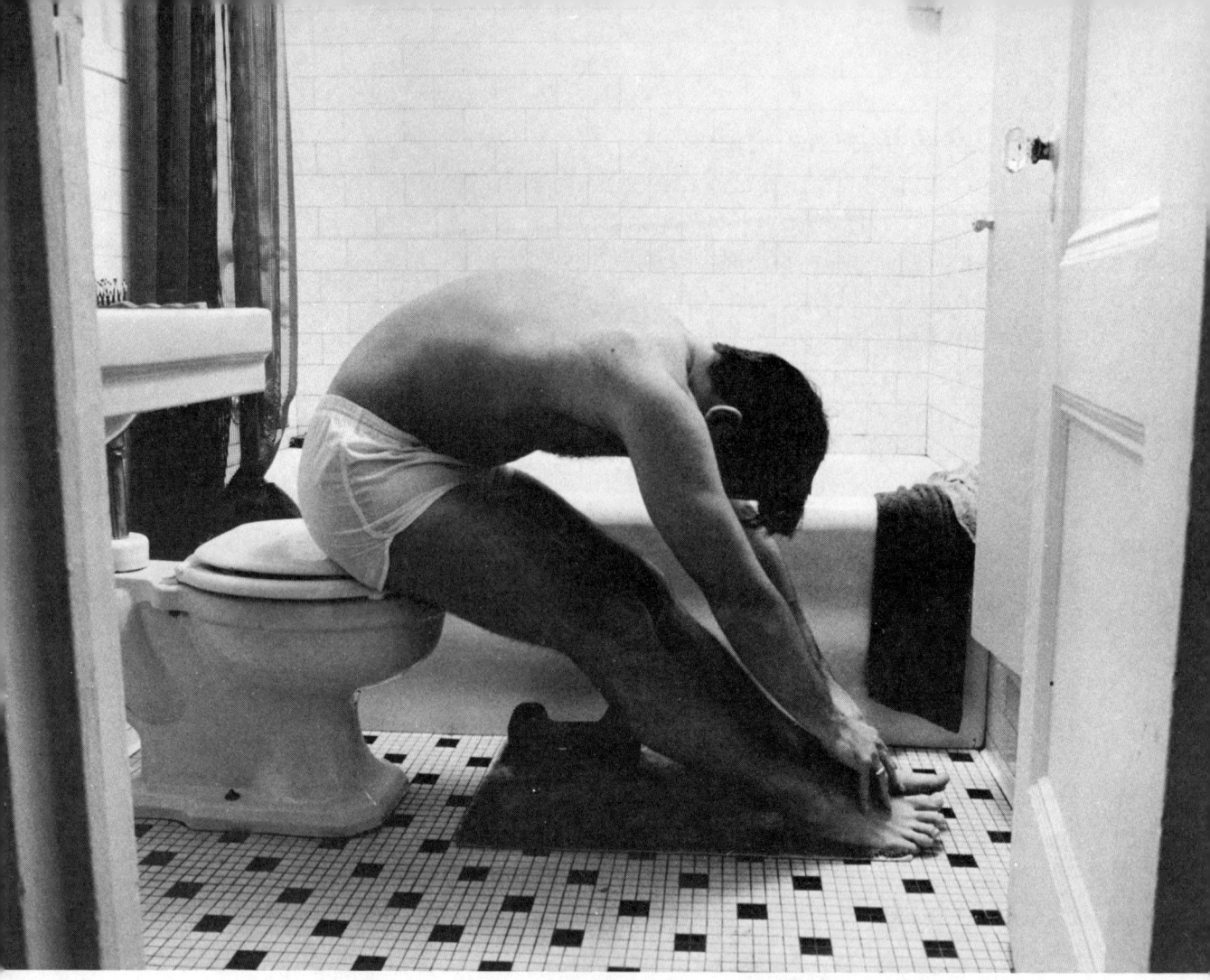

The best feeling after your morning shower is a good stretch.

- When you tan naturally, some parts of your face get more than others. After applying bronzer to your entire face, go back and put just a bit more on your cheekbones, forehead, nose, and chin. You don't need to put any bronzer on areas that would usually not get sun—the eyelids and behind the ears.
- You can get the bronzer off your fingers by washing with soap and water. Use a toner to remove stubborn spots.
- Always remove bronzer before going to bed. If your usual soap and water washing doesn't completely remove all traces, clean your skin with a toner. Moisturize as usual.

Concealers

When no amount of basic skin care can cover up the dark circles under your eyes after a long night or the occasional blemish that pops us unannounced, you can grab a quick cover-up called a concealer.

Concealers are skin-toned in light, medium, medium dark, and dark shades and come in retractable "stick" containers. When you need to cover up a pimple or dark circle, you just smooth on the concealer and blend it into your skin with your fingers. You can pick up a concealer like Erase by Max Factor in any drugstore, and no one will be the wiser.

Just as proper hair care takes a bit more time, making your skin radiate health takes some extra effort. I think it's worth it. Not only are you improving your appearance, you're taking some positive steps to keep your skin healthier and younger-looking longer.

Great skin and great hair—they're two of the best things you can give yourself.

Now you know what women have known for years: Hair is a strong point for your good looks. Use it to your advantage to project your best image. The men in this book are bankers, lawyers, actors; some are famous, some are not. Each has his own unique hair and facial characteristics. Each has put all his special components together to create a look that is custom-designed to suit his work and his way of life and versatile enough to adapt to all the things he wants to do and be. I hope this book will guide you to do the same.

Index